MORE

More is a daring and inspirational memoir offering the reader the opportunity to experience the potential for healing and enlightenment from the inside out as you go with Mariah on a journey of self-discovery that begins when she and her husband participate in my yearlong Love and Ecstasy Training. Mariah's memoir offers a ray of light both to individuals and to couples. Her work will appeal to a large audience.

Margot Anand, SkyDancing Tantra founder and author of *The Art of Sexual Ecstasy*

More is just as the title promises. It is much more than a journey of a woman and man finding healing through sexual intimacy, orgasmic pleasure and sensual adventure, all of which it includes. It is the journey of a human spirit moving to inner peace with herself so she can find divine union with another. It is more than a self-help book. *More* is a book of transcendence that speaks to all people as we attempt to rise above our fears and traumas to our higher selves.

Asra Q. Nomani, former *Wall Street Journal* reporter and author of *Tantrika: Traveling the Road of Divine Love*

Here is a bold celebration of holy intimacy and its capacity to heal. Kudos to McKenzie for her courage to share this story!

Elizabeth Jarrett Andrew, author of *Writing the Sacred Journey*

I heartily endorse Mariah's story of her spiritual journey. It has all the features that make a compelling spiritual autobiography as well as those that make a touching love story. There is soul-searching, despair and its transcendence as well as heart-wrenching desire and its fulfillment. Mariah and her husband have committed themselves to the spiritual path as well as to each other with commendable tenacity. And the juicy bits are sure to turn the properly prudish red with embarrassment or perhaps green with envy. I highly recommend this book to anyone trying to balance busy lives with meditation practice, and especially to anyone seeking to heal from sexual trauma and transform their lives in the pursuit of highest Love.

Matthew Sieradski, Spiritual Teacher, Center for Sacred Sciences

Mariah's story of love and spiritual transformation will not only grab your heart but will challenge you to think of the way you view love, sexuality and spiritual fulfillment in ways you probably have not done before. It's the story for every busy mom who thinks she has no time for spirituality or sexuality. It's the story for anyone who has experienced trauma or shame and wonders if they can be fully sexual and love with a full heart. It's the story for anyone who yearns for more but fears they cannot pursue their deepest dreams. Mariah's seductive and beautifully written tale gives us all the permission we need to begin our own search for "more."

Marni Freedman, Therapist, Professor of Writing, Playwright

More

Journey to mystical union through
the sacred and the profane

More

Journey to mystical union through
the sacred and the profane

Mariah McKenzie

BOOKS

Winchester, UK
Washington, USA

First published by O-Books, 2016
O-Books is an imprint of John Hunt Publishing Ltd., Laurel House, Station Approach,
Alresford, Hants, SO24 9JH, UK
office1@jhpbooks.net
www.johnhuntpublishing.com

For distributor details and how to order please visit the 'Ordering' section on our website.

Text copyright: Mariah McKenzie 2015

ISBN: 978 1 78535 262 1
Library of Congress Control Number: 2015949723

A CIP catalogue record for this book is available from the British Library.

Permissions:
From the Penguin publication *The Purity of Desire: 100 Poems of Rumi*. Copyright © 2012 Daniel
Ladinsky and used with his permission.

From the Penguin publication *The Gift: Poems by Hafiz*. Copyright © 1999 Daniel Ladinsky and
used with his permission.

Publisher's Note:
Some names and identifying details have been changed to protect the privacy of individuals.

Design: Stuart Davies

Printed and bound by CPI Group (UK) Ltd, Croydon, CR0 4YY, UK

We operate a distinctive and ethical publishing philosophy in all
areas of our business, from our global network of authors to
production and worldwide distribution.

CONTENTS

Dedicated to My Beloved Rudra

This is a wake-up call; the events in your life are trying to show you a pattern as ancient as the journey of your own soul.

~ Osho

In Gratitude

Thank you to San Diego Writer's Ink for hosting the 2012 Fall for Writing Conference, and to Judy Reeves for teaching a "Show, Don't Tell" workshop that enticed me to begin writing again after an 18-year hiatus. After stepping into Judy Reeve's workshop, I fell back in love with the whole writing process. Everything stilled in that room and I noted the fluttering of the leaves behind the leaded glass windows. I noted Judy Reeves' short hair, pointy cowboy boots and infectious easy laugh and I remembered what I love about writing—it brings me precisely to the present moment, paying attention and appreciating everything.

Thank you also to Judy Reeves for pointing to the back of the room that day and introducing Marni Freedman. Marni, she said, was a great resource for non-fiction writers. I was thinking about writing a cooking blog, so I made it a point to introduce myself. What I didn't know at the time is that I would be writing a spiritual memoir instead and that Marni would become my writing coach/therapist and good friend—someone I could trust with my baby when it was newly born. Truthfully, this memoir would not have been written without her support and encouragement not only for the writing, but for the in-between moments when I struggled emotionally, when I doubted myself, when I shied away from the hard truths. Marni's Memoir Club also provided a safe place for me and my fellow memoirists to practice sharing our personal stories and to learn together how to structure them for the enjoyment of others. I am deeply grateful to her. An appreciative nod also to Tracy Jones for her reading of a very early draft. Her comments led to important restructuring.

A happy thank-you too to the Alpine Writers Guild, in particular Catherine, Marla, Shirley, and Teresa for helping me hone key chapters of the memoir and for working on endless drafts of my synopsis. A special thank-you to Marla for being the first advanced reader of the pre-edited manuscript and offering key advice before I turned it over to Shirley Clukey for copyediting. Shirley's gentle, respectful, yet spot-on copyediting turned the manuscript into a real book and I am deeply grateful for her invaluable service and also for her friendship.

A deep *gassho* to Durga, my friend, confidante, and fellow spiritual wayfarer, who has always been there for me, offering love and compassion, turning my attention back to the Truth, back to the Source. Durga once told me the highest aspiration in life is to be a good friend. That she is. Durga has seen the good, the bad, and the ugly and always remained a friend, regardless of distance or circumstance.

Finally, to my beloved husband Rudra, who has lived this entire sacred and profane journey with me, and with whom I have touched the infinite, a deep bow: "I honor you, Rudra, as an aspect of myself." In the moments when I realize that if there is no "I" there is no "we" either, I have fallen apart. But you, Rudra, in your inimitable way gently remind me there is always an "us." Thank you for holding my hand along the way.

Part I

The Doorway

It began with a distinct urgent need to go home immediately—a feeling so strong and compelling I at once turned to the young man sitting next to me, whom I knew only as a minor acquaintance, and asked if I could borrow his truck. He looked at me strangely, but must have seen the panic in my eyes and agreed. I snatched the keys from him and ran out of the writer's conference. I drove straight home, and pulled into my driveway with heart pounding.

What happened next changed the course and direction of my life. It was a course correction that ultimately did lead me home—a home that I discovered was not a physical place, but the deepest inviolable core of my heart.

Chapter 1

Kindred Spirits

Back to the beginning . . .

It was a rare hot day in Bellingham, Washington, the day I met Jake in the summer of 1981. I pulled into the parking lot of my apartment relieved to be home. The weekend had been hectic as the younger 17-year-old brother of a friend had contacted me and asked if I'd take him and his buddies on a tour of the university and town. I had spent the last half-day driving them around in a loud, old, non-air-conditioned Mustang, with the music blaring. I dripped with sweat and felt cranky after having been stuffed between two immature, boisterous teenage boys in the back seat—uggh. I was happy to have done my duty and to be home. They pulled up and I clambered out clumsily from the low-slung vehicle, hailing a goodbye to them as they peeled out laughing and singing, barely noticing I had left.

I readjusted my bikini top, which was somewhat askew after my escape from the teen-boy-mobile, finger combed my thick, wavy, shoulder-length brown hair, then looked up and saw another car in the parking lot. My friend, Debbie, who lived in the same apartment complex as me, was standing by the car and motioned to me to come over. I walked to the car, saw her parents in the front seat, and hailed a warm greeting. Debbie introduced me to her brother, Jake, sitting in the back, and I found myself falling into the most beautiful blue eyes in the world, set in a tanned face surrounded by tight blond curls. I forgot Debbie had mentioned to me that her brother—someone she briefly described as "a 4.0 engineering-frat-boy from

UCLA"—was going to be visiting that summer. I had written him off before meeting him, thinking he was out of my league and never imagining that I could be attracted to a frat boy. His compelling presence took me by surprise. I would find out later he wasn't at all what his sister's description implied with the frat boy label—neither overly preppy, nor overly *Animal House* rambunctious. No, he chose his fraternity for practical reasons: it was located close to the university and he was able to barter dishwashing services in exchange for room and board—an important consideration while putting himself through college. Years later, wondering if it was love at first sight for him too, I asked him what he'd thought when he first saw me that day.

"Ha!" he said chuckling. "When I saw you climb out of that car full of guys that day, half falling out of your bikini, I thought you were either taken . . . or a hussy!"

I was flabbergasted, but also secretly pleased. At the time, although not a virgin, I was rather naive and self-conscious, and identified more with being a dedicated student and outdoor adventure type than a party girl. Actually, I worried about being five pounds too heavy to be considered "sexy." Thus, despite the fact that I was wearing a bikini top (as were all the college girls that hot July day), it never occurred to me that I could come off that way.

Thankfully, I had another chance to make a better impression a few days later, when he and his parents came to eat at the restaurant where his sister and I worked. That night I was dressed up to be hostess for the evening and had the chance to escort them to their table. His sister and I had just come up with the idea of going dancing in Vancouver, British Columbia, and we invited him along as an escort.

A few days later, on a crowded dance floor, Jake and I gazed into one another's eyes while we danced for hours and the rest of the world slipped away, leaving only each other at the center. At last, I inwardly sighed, a guy who likes to dance. I was so sick of hanging out with guys who didn't like to do *anything* except sit around drinking, smoking, and listening to music.

A little over a month later, now officially dating, we lay on our backs on sleeping bags set on the cool grass in his parents' backyard on Lummi Island. The embers of our bonfire were still burning, as though ready to ignite our new friendship into something more. We gazed together into the endless, dark, night sky, exclaiming with wonder and delight at a multitude of shooting stars—courtesy of the Perseid meteor shower. Staring into infinity with him, I remembered being a small child, looking up into the sky and seeing my first rainbow, spell-struck by the unexpected mystery and beauty of that sight.

"Let's travel together," Jake whispered to me under the stars.

"Okay. Where should we go?" I whispered back, giggling.

"How about Mexico? Let's drive to the Yucatan."

My heart leapt out of my chest. I loved the idea.

"Really? Is that possible?"

"Sure, why not?"

"You mean now? This summer?"

"Well, we might not make it that far this summer," he said with a twinkle in his eye, "but we can get to Mexico, for sure. And we can drive and camp through Yosemite and the Grand Canyon on the way."

"Oh Jake. I would sooooo love to do that." My 20-year-old bohemian pixie self was tickled with the thought that I might have found a smart, dancing, adventuring, kindred soul to play with. I felt an opening in my tremulous heart. Maybe this was the man for me . . .

The next day we decided to take a long walk with his sister down the western shore of Lummi. The beach was strewn with rocks, driftwood, and kelp; tiny bits of sea glass peppered the walk along with miscellaneous flotsam and jetsam. The frigid Puget Sound quietly lapped the shore; on the cliffs above, tall evergreen trees stood sentinel the whole way. Occasionally we would hear the chattering cries of a couple of bald eagles who frequented the area.

The three of us walked for miles down the beach, happy and unconcerned. At the far end a gathering of tiny islands called "Lummi Rocks" rested a half-mile offshore.

Jake looked longingly over at them. "I've always wanted to go out there," he said.

He stood looking out to sea for a moment, and then turned his attention back to the beach.

"Hey, I know," he said. "Let's build a raft. Right here. Right now. We can have our picnic out there." He pointed to the little island and his eyes sparkled with fun and delight at the prospect.

"A raft?" I said. "How are we going to build a raft?"

I looked around at the deserted stretch of coast and mentally considered what we had brought along in our daypack that might help . . . a knife, a fork?

"We'll have to gather big pieces of driftwood," he said slowly, and then added enthusiastically, "and we can tie them together with pieces of bull kelp."

Make a raft out of driftwood and kelp? How exciting! What fun!

"I don't want to do that," his sister said, a look of terror passing over her face. My heart fell for a minute. "But you two go ahead. I'll wait here," she added quickly. It seemed sort of mean to leave her out, but I couldn't resist the thrill of it. She smiled and encouraged us. "It's better this way in case you need someone back on shore to rescue you."

Jake and I began searching for just the right pieces, leaving behind all thoughts of the dangers and foolhardiness of trying to build a raft seaworthy enough to cross the expanse of water to Lummi Rocks. I mean anyone who lives in Washington State learns to appreciate the potential for hypothermia if you swim unprotected in the Puget Sound for more than 20 minutes or so. What if the raft fell apart half way? But that was not our focus.

Instead Jake and I were on the same wavelength: little kids playing, exploring, about to embark on an uncharted adventure. Westward Ho!

We hauled the biggest logs we could find and lined them up in rows, tying them together, as Jake had suggested, with pieces of kelp. We put two strong brace logs crosswise underneath and tied those on too.

Jake tested the knots. They held. We pushed our contraption to the water's edge.

"Okay," Jake said gamely. "Let's set sail."

"Wait," I cried, running up the beach. I came back triumphantly carrying two additional pieces of wood. "Our paddles," I said, grinning, climbing on board.

We felt our raft begin to float and we began paddling away from shore, our legs straddled over the logs, dangling in the water.

Midway across, it got pretty scary. The current pulled us along, and eddies haphazardly circled our raft. I felt a little nervous and could see Jake's furrowed brows as he appraised the situation.

"We have to paddle harder," he said. "We need to make sure we stay in the lee of the island. We don't want to get swept around the corner of Lummi Rocks into the open Sound."

"Should we turn back?" I asked Jake.

"We could," he said. "What do you think?"

I paused, considering. "Let's see if we can make it."

We kept on, now paddling harder, and began to make headway again; the tiny island grew closer. We selected a landing spot and just as we were making our way in, a large wave came and threw us hard onto the rocks. I managed to grab our backpack, just as it came untied and began sliding off the raft. We heard something shatter.

"Oh! Our wine!" we cried together.

We pulled our rickety, though still intact craft up onto a rock as best we could and awkwardly clambered ashore, unable to walk properly at first because our legs were so numb from the freezing water.

Standing on our conquered shore, we waved back at his sister, turned and grinned gleefully at each other, "We made it."

In that moment with that man, it seemed anything might be possible. Life stretched before us as one grand adventure and I sensed that we might have found in each other a companion to share the way, however foolhardy and rough it got.

At the end of that summer Jake had to return to LA where he was at school. We talked on the phone and sent cards and letters to one another that fall, then I flew down to be with him for Christmas. Jake picked me up at the airport in an old, red Triumph sports car that he had spent months getting to run. It was super-cute and romantic, but what I remember most about the drive back to his place was the silence. Even at the time I noted it was unusual that, although we barely knew each other, the silence between us was comfortable rather than awkward. Within a month, I had moved to Los Angeles and changed schools.

Four years after we met, we got married in a small glass church called "The Wayfarer's Chapel," perched high on a bluff overlooking the Pacific Ocean in Rancho Palos Verde, California—still the hero and pixie of our own fairytale. We continued to fill our life with adventure: backpacking through Europe on a shoestring, walking 450 miles from San Francisco to the Oregon border, and yes, as promised, eventually driving to the Yucatan and back in an old, mustard yellow pickup truck with a bright orange wood canopy. Five years later, we embarked on an adventure of a different kind, when we decided to have children. We moved back to Washington State, where our parents lived, and were blessed with two tow-headed, sweet girls.

Still, we made time for one another. One night when we'd been contemplating the meaning of life and love, Jake whispered to me in the darkness, "It's easy to overlook the obvious. After twelve years you still excite me. I lust after you. You turn me on. That is something rare and real—a foundation to grow on—even if it goes against the grain to think of life in terms of sex."

I turned that thought over in my mind, wondering about all the things I had read about sex not having to be the basis of marriage. But I reflected on all the closeness we had felt and concluded that if there was one thing I couldn't bear to live without, it was our hot steamy nights—our unbridled passion, his eagerness always—the dark, rich passages we had traveled together in heated, wild moments of ecstasy.

Some would say—I would say—that we lived a dream life and a juicy one at that. Nevertheless, there was a growing feeling within me that one day the other shoe would drop. I realized that our love had never been tested. Fear began to grow inside me insidiously. I feared death. I feared the unknown. Mostly, I feared losing Jake. I felt like we had a precious thing and I wanted desperately to control our destiny—to keep our fairytale life intact. I didn't know the source of my fear, although I had begun to realize that Jake suffered from bouts of depression, probably genetic and certainly compounded by the gray Pacific Northwest weather.

In the fall of 1994, the other shoe did begin to slip, slowly at first, with my dawning awareness that Jake was stuck in a deep, mostly work-related depression. He stopped responding to my efforts to cheer him up, leaving me feeling powerless and scared. I should be able to help him. Where is he? I need him!

I missed him terribly during his bouts of depression. My sense of being alone and helpless compounded my fear, which grew and started to present itself as anxiety attacks.

I hated to let Jake out of my sight, to be apart from him. I recognized I wasn't like the other wives, who welcomed a day off from their guy. I wanted to be with him every moment. I wanted to hold him back, to keep him home, to keep him safe. Also, truthfully, I wanted my hero to be available to protect *me*—from what I wasn't sure. I only knew that I felt secure in his arms.

A growing series of "what ifs?" began to control me. What if something happened to Jake? What if he died?

In less than a year, we were in a tailspin careening toward a crisis—a crisis that tested our love and forced me to face "what ifs" I had never before considered: What if Jake falls into a depression and doesn't come out? What if Jake doesn't want to be with me? What if we are broken? What if I am not enough?

Soon, we would desperately need something more.

Chapter 2

Dreams

In rare cases a dream with an exceptionally strong archetypal content can itself precipitate an abrupt shift from worldly to spiritual seeking . . .

~ Joel Morwood

It turns out "more" was on the horizon—just not the more I had imagined. It all started in October 1994 when an article I had written for *Woman's Day* about Jake and me having "dancing dates" caught the attention of a Seattle morning news television program director. She contacted me about a piece she wanted to do on us that featured our dancing life along with a live interview. I was thrilled. I talked to Jake about it; he seemed a little nervous, but tentatively agreed. It turns out this was his idea of hell, and the stress of anticipating being on TV precipitated an anxiety attack that actually landed him in the hospital a few days before the event. We almost canceled. At the last moment, probably because the director told me I could come on the show alone, Jake got better and decided to come along.

In the dressing room of the television station the following morning, we were telling the makeup lady how he had been in the hospital the day before. She explained that she used to get nervous like that before she took up Zen Buddhism and started to meditate. She recommended a book to us titled *Zen Mind, Beginner's Mind*, by Shunryu Suzuki.

It's funny how you never realize the moment when someone unwittingly launches you on a trajectory that will change your life. This small, but definitive moment was the beginning of a journey ultimately beset with dreams, coincidences, and signposts guiding us out of the dark. But not before things got much darker.

Jake's depression worsened that winter and I felt more and more helpless. Nothing I did seemed to cheer him up. Finally, I decided that we should take an extended family vacation to La Paz, Baja California. Baja had been the source of great fun and adventure for us when we were first married. While we had plenty of family activities in mind, and I hoped to write a travel article out of our trip, we also planned to carve out some time for each other. The hotel we were staying at had babysitters available. We planned to get away for a mini-adventure of climbing a local mountain at sunrise one day, and then thought we'd try to steal away for a night dancing with each other. I was looking forward to it all and hoped the getaway would be good for Jake.

Unfortunately, the trip started out a little rocky. As the plane took off, my heart began beating wildly and I was terrified. I grabbed Jake's hand, squeezing it until it was blue, trying not to shake in front of the children, who were seated next to us. Inwardly, I began to pay hyper-attention to every little sound the plane was making, and kept glancing out the window at the wings and engines, convinced something was wrong. I became acutely aware of my lack of control over the destiny of that flight; it caused me great anxiety. I couldn't help but think how ironic it was that just as I was becoming successful as a travel writer, my fear of flying was growing worse.

One night while we were on vacation in La Paz, I struck up a conversation in the hotel bar with a man named Mark. During margaritas on the rocks and a "Lion King" sunset, Mark told me he saw life as a series of patterns and that it was important to pay attention to coincidences or synchronicities, because they could guide you. He also told me he was a Buddhist, which caught my attention because of the interaction with the makeup lady. He said he did not fear death—that he saw it only as a transition. That intrigued me. I told him I was afraid of dying, or of someone close to me dying, and that I'd developed an almost paralyzing fear of flying.

"That's interesting—and coincidental," he said, winking. "As it turns out my job is to run and maintain flight simulators for the airlines. Why don't you and your husband come over and try it out? Maybe it will help you get over your fear."

We met him the next night out in the desert, at a warehouse where the flight simulator was housed. Jake went first and was super-excited to successfully land a 737 in the program. I tried too, strapping myself into the real pilot's seat before a working console. The experience was incredibly lifelike. The floor pitched and rolled like a real airplane as you managed the controls, while a video simulated the visual and sound effects of landing. Unfortunately, I developed an anxiety attack much like those I get when flying for real and choked while simulating the landing. Had I actually been piloting the plane, we would have crashed. Ultimately, I felt even more scared and ill-prepared to face death; the event made me realize how dependent I was on Jake to keep me safe.

Then, the night after our experience in the flight simulator, Jake and I both had extraordinarily intense dreams—top five in a lifetime type. Mine involved knowing my death was near. In the years to come I would have several significant dreams, all involving my death. In this one, I only needed one-third of a bottle of water for the rest of my life. As I started drinking it, someone asked me what plans I'd made for death and I panicked and sobbed into wakefulness. I tried to wake Jake, who soothingly shushed me, saying everything would be all right, but it didn't feel all right. I got out of bed, and huddling on the patio outside the hotel room, I wrote in my journal:

Jake – I trust you more than I trust myself. Is this a weak moment? I am weak. I am curious about Buddhism. Sitting here on the patio hallway shortly after my dream, you are a few feet away inside. I need your kind words. You always have kind words.

(Journal entry, March 1995)

In the morning I wanted to talk to Jake about my dream, but he woke up restless and agitated.

"What's up, Jake?" I asked, wanting a chance to talk to him.

"I had a dream . . . " he started. "It was amazing. I am still tingling . . . "

"Wow, cool!" I said, but actually wanted to get to the part where I talked to him about my dream. "I had an intense dream too," I said. "Mine was really scary. There were these death vendors, and—"

He looked at me strangely. "No, really," he said. "I think it was an important dream somehow. I feel weird. In the dream, this woman came to me. She was standing on a shell . . . I think it was the goddess Venus," he said slowly. "She placed hot rocks on my back and then sang to me, 'Turn around, bright eyes.' You know from that song—what's it called, oh yeah: 'Total Eclipse of the Heart.' I know that sounds kind of corny, but the important part was that she was telling me to turn around. I think she was telling me to wake up—you know, to transcend this reality, like in Carlos Castaneda's books!" Jake sat there for a minute, obviously consumed by his dream.

He turned to me, his eyes clear and piercing, and said, "I think that was the most powerful experience of bliss I have ever had! My whole body was ringing from head to toe."

I tried to wrap my head around what he was saying. Waking up? Bliss? Hot rocks? Some woman singing to him? I was still fearing death from my own dream, filled with anxiety, and I needed to talk more, but it was too late, the kids were waking up.

Jake got up and began cuddling and dressing our two- and five-year-old girls.

I sat there. Even without knowing the future, in that moment his dream scared me almost as much as my own. I felt small and jealous. *I* wanted to be the source of the deepest bliss he had ever had. Who was this woman in his dream?

I got up and we all made our way outside. I was still feeling anxious and worried, but we had promised the kids a day at the pool. Thankfully, we had scheduled our dancing date for that night. I figured we would have a chance to talk then. And, if we didn't have the chance tonight, I thought, we could always bond while climbing the mountain together, which we had yet to do. For the moment, I planned to forget about our dreams and escape in a pool lounge chair by diving into my John Grisham book and watching the kids play. Jake, however, was still agitated from his dream and couldn't settle down. He stopped by my pool lounger.

"Hey, I think I'm just going to take a walk, okay?"

"Sure," I said. "I'll watch the kids."

Jake took off and was gone for several hours. In the afternoon, I took a long soak and got dolled up in my sexiest dress for our date. Finally, a night out together.

"I'm tired," Jake said, once we were in town.

"Tired?" I asked, rather incredulous that my husband would even consider thinking about being tired on such a special occasion. "You're . . . tired? I thought we were going dancing."

"Yeah, well . . . " he said, pausing, "I climbed the mountain today."

I stopped still. The words echoed in my head. The mountain? It was as if he had slapped me in the face. But climbing the mountain was the sunrise date we had planned. Climbing the mountain was the challenge we were doing together. Climbing the mountain . . . was sacred.

We ended up getting in one of the worst fights of our

relationship.

I just couldn't wrap my head around it. Questions kept circling: Why had he climbed the mountain alone? Why did his dream have such an impact on him? Would this woman from his dream come between us? Something was nagging at me—it seemed like something worse was on the horizon.

Chapter 3

Seduction

These tumultuous feelings. I keep looking for boundaries wondering about love. What defines our love? Keeps it special? Makes it sacred? What is the difference between true love and possession? What path are we all heading down? Am I too controlling or not enough? This feeling is similar to my fear of flying. My heart is pounding, chest constricted, mind flying over possibilities over which I have no control.
~ Journal entry, early summer 1995

The sun was shining brightly on Lummi Island that early July day in 1995 a few months after returning from our vacation in La Paz: fir trees and falcons were magnificently set off against the sparkling Puget Sound; in the distance other islands making up the San Juan archipelago beckoned us hither.

Jake and I and our daughters, Jacki and Cassie, had come up to the family cottage with our good friends, Shari and Greg, and their two kids, a boy and a girl roughly the same age as our girls. For the last year or so, we had been developing a friendship with them that had grown steadily closer. I was pleased to have a girlfriend, as it had always been harder for me to make friends with girls than guys. It helped that we all were in the same stage of life, I guess, trying to juggle parenting and work with fun, play, and a little adventure.

We had begun gathering regularly at one or the other's house almost every weekend. The 30-something adults would party in one room, while the kids would play in another. We'd play loud music and dance and often ended up imbibing in the hot tub. During these raucous get-togethers we let loose, perhaps too much, drinking to excess and becoming increasingly flirty and coquettish with one another. As time went on, it became more difficult to constrain those feelings within acceptable social bounds. It was like we were all in heat.

Shari was beautiful, a cross between Jane Seymour and Keira Knightley, with big eyes and long brown hair that hung down her back, soft bangs across her forehead. I envied her tight, lithe figure, seeing it as everything my softer, more voluptuous body was not. She could wear short shorts and men would still whistle at her in the streets. She was also a lovely, patient, and kind mother, who sang sweet lullabies to her children every night. Still, there was something else about her that was more difficult to pinpoint. We played a game one night with our husbands where we had to use one word to describe each one of us. The word we chose for Shari was "strategic." She told me once that her mother had committed suicide when she was about four years old and I wondered what that did to a person. I think I flattered myself that she needed me.

One day prior to the weekend at Lummi, Shari came over. We had decided to undertake a new workout routine that included using Jake's home weight-lifting set.

"What should we wear?" we giggled, as we modeled our athletic attire for one another, proud that we had each kept in shape after the birth of our children. We went into the garage where the equipment was set up and began lifting weights. We were sweating and grunting and generally making fun of ourselves in a lighthearted way, but there was an undercurrent of something else. Shari broached the subject first.

"I just don't know what to do with all these sexual feelings!" she laughed.

"Well, isn't the saying supposed to be that you can have

feelings, but you just don't act on them? Isn't that something they taught you for your work as a therapist?"

"I know," she said panting heavily, "but they are just so strong! I've got crazy hormones."

Still, as 30-somethings living in Issaquah, Washington during the 1990s, from most perspectives we were respectable grown-ups with good jobs, well-versed in the benefits of organic food, and religiously practicing "positive parenting." We had an expert in the group as Shari's training had been in Human Development and Family Studies prior to quitting her work to raise her children. She kept us informed as to the latest theories.

"Remember," she'd say. "You can discipline with natural consequences rather than arbitrary ones. If your kid colors on the floor, the natural consequence is not to put them into time out, but to have them scrub the floor clean."

I appreciated her wisdom and tried out her techniques regularly, laughing and reporting back to her when they didn't work.

"So," I reported one day. "I tried the self-esteem booster. You know the one where you are supposed to ask your kid about the picture instead of interpreting it? Well, I saw Jacki coloring the other day and I couldn't figure out what she was drawing, so I said 'What can you tell me about your picture, honey?' like you were telling us. Jacki turned around and looked at me with a funny look on her face and said, 'It's a scribble, Mommy.' Hah! I felt like an idiot!" I said, and we had a good chuckle.

On Lummi that weekend some time later, from the balcony of the family cottage, nicknamed "The Cliff House," Shari and I watched otters swim and neighbors' dogs frolic and listened to snatches caught on the wind of our children playing pirate on huge pieces of driftwood scattered over the pebbly beach below. By midmorning that first day, the grown-ups all decided to hike up the mountain with the kids. On the way up, we found a scenic bluff from which we could sit and eat up the view along with our snacks. Lying directly before us, Orcas Island dominated the scene. Mammoth and humped, it was an Orca itself. At its north end, the nearby, smaller islands of Clark and Barnes appeared to swim, babies hanging close to Mom. Further in the distance Sucia and Matia snuggled together.

The guys were pumped, dreams of bushwhacking to the peak motivating them. For a moment we considered all going, but there was no trail and the children were already tired. Before the rest of us realized what had happened, Greg and Jake had taken off on their manly quest. Shari and I explored our immediate surroundings. The six-year-olds dared each other to rock climb up a nearby hillside, safe from the cliff's edge. The three-year-olds found a secret hiding place within the dense shrubbery.

After a while, we moms and kids prepared to go back down the trail to the cliff house, leaving an arrow of sticks and a heart made of wild flowers and twigs for the daddies to show we'd gone down. But Greg and Jake arrived before we finished, vibrating with the energy of their adventure. They came from the mountain like men in a Conan book, bare-chested, long hair flowing, bearing huge bush-beating sticks and scars from their adventure. They were breathless as they told us of climbing over ridges and beating back nettle fields and finding at last a grassy knoll at the peak.

"You must go," Greg told us.

There was still plenty of daylight left. I looked at Shari, sensing fun and adventure. Would we make it to the top? Were we worthy women for such men?

The guys left us with instructions: "Take a left at the pink-ribboned shale pit, then head south over several ridges until you get to the peak. Take our sticks too. You'll need them."

We headed up the trail full of he-woman energy, yet giddy. We were a couple of young girl scouts out after dark, behind the counselors' backs.

At the shale pit, we looked left. The mountainside rose

steadily from the road. There was no trail. Clambering over moss-covered rocks and dead branches, we conquered the hillside. The climb energized me even more. Small, dead pieces of twigs clung to Shari's and my hair, cobwebs laced our shorts, branches scratched our bare arms and legs. The air smelled fresh of fir trees mingled with wild black raspberries and stinging nettles. I clambered up the next set of boulders and walked briskly through the forest to a resting spot between two tall trees. Another set of boulders loomed before us. My legs pumped. I breathed deep as Shari and I beamed at each other. God, it was great to be alive.

By chance at that moment I looked down and caught my breath. There at my feet rested a perfect deer antler. Its base rose into two Pan-like horns. In the magic of the moment I felt the mountain calling to me, saying, "Yes, it is a gift for you. A special gift; you must treasure it and appreciate it. You have been chosen."

"Shari, look," I whispered, picking it up. "Isn't it beautiful?" We stood and gazed at it in awe, handling it carefully, turning it over, feeling the gentle curve of the horns. Then in an instant I saw another just ahead of Shari on her path.

Standing there on the mountainside away from any man-made trails, we felt the sacredness of the moment. We held our antlers together, in reverence.

I read sometime later that the deer symbolizes innocence and unconditional love; the antlers are said to be antennae to the divine. Shamanic traditions teach that deer lure a person to new adventures to gain more wisdom, and that while one should not be afraid to follow, one should stay alert, for adventurous journeys are not always without danger. I did not know it at the time, but this innocent and sweet moment marked a transition point, after which I would never be the same.

We found the grassy knoll of the peak, peeled off our tops like the guys, and stood for several minutes in shock at the beauty.

Before us stretched all the San Juan Islands. There was Cypress and San Juan. We could look behind Orcas now. We stood there on our cliff, staffs in one hand, horns in the other, bare-chested, proud women.

The sun on the cliff side was intoxicating. We stripped completely nude just to enjoy the sensation of sunbathing on a mountaintop. We picked up the phallic antlers, each of which had a rough base about one and a half inches in diameter and rose up about six inches before splitting into two sections that made a curved "Y." We fondled them as if they were men and joked about what we could do with them. After a bit, we agreed it must be time to go.

"You know what I'm going to do, Shari?" I teased, as we donned our cut-offs.

"What?" she said, eyes dancing.

"I'm going to rest the base of the antler down in my shorts with the horns facing up, so that each horn rests against the crease of my groins. See, it makes a perfect curved Y, nestled in the crotch of my shorts. I'm going to hike down the mountain that way. "

Shari giggled and tried out hers as well. We dressed, but left our tops off; they felt too cumbersome.

"This is exquisite," she crooned.

"Yes," I said in a husky voice, "isn't it?"

What a hike down the mountain that was. We were keyed up and quite, well . . . horny. Yeah, we laughed at that too. With each step, the rough end of the base of the horn grazed the lips of my nether regions. If I walked with a little sway I found I could keep the stimulation high.

Shari and I were giddy, like two of Pan's wood nymphs: simple sprites of the mountain.

Half way down, we rested in a grassy glen under a willow tree. We lay on our backs, arms barely touching, and watched the wind blow the leaves. We watched the leaves flutter and whisper to each other in the breeze and listened to the quiet sounds of the mountain. We whispered to each other, too.

"Isn't this nice," Shari said dreamily. "It's been hard lately at home . . ."

"Oh, I'm so sorry," I said gently.

Shari's husband, Greg, was a brilliant cancer researcher who had resisted getting a lucrative job with a biogenetic company and remained in academia because of his principles, but it paid little and required long hours in the lab. Shari and Greg were having a hard time and usually she tried to joke about it.

"It pretty much sucks," she'd say. "He's never home and his job pays so little I have to go to the food bank for food and clothes for the kids! I wish I could get really mad and say 'It's not like he's curing cancer or something!' but I can't, because he is ..."

I offered some empathy. "Jake's been having a hard time too, you know. Since the elite High Technology Center of Boeing closed, he's been shuffled off to some other department and has to commute 45 minutes. Jobs in his area are hard to come by. I know he is unhappy and feels trapped by his responsibilities, but I feel helpless as to how to help him, what with our mortgage and all."

Shari knew Jake had been depressed, but we hadn't talked about what exactly had been going on for him. In the years since Jake and I had met, he had become a creative and innovative engineer who had authored nine patents. Presently, he was supremely frustrated with his work situation, having grown increasingly despondent over the last year. He had started getting sick a lot. A California boy at heart, the typically dreary, drippy Pacific Northwest weather was seriously affecting him. He looked like a poster boy for seasonal affective disorder (SAD).

But Shari didn't see that side of him. We mostly saw each other in a party atmosphere. I had taken to inviting Shari and some other girlfriends to our house in the afternoon. We set up crafts for the kids and got them busy playing. Then we girls would play dress-up. Jake, who rarely worked late these days, would come home to find the gathering of women at our house. We'd be dressed up in some sort of outlandish costume, music blaring when he opened the door. There is a photo of us, taken during one of these sessions, that Jake kept in his briefcase for years. In it, I am wearing a low-cut sheer bodice top, a red lace-up corset and see-through pants. Kate is lifting a glass of wine to the camera, and Shari and Corine, in short shorts, long hair swinging free, are leaning in close to my breasts, grinning at the camera, which was wielded by Jake. Jake and his harem . . .

I felt a little sorry for Greg sometimes, missing out on the fun so often. Sometimes, after meeting with my editor in Seattle, I would stop by Greg's research lab to say hi, and see what he was up to. It was my way of trying to keep him involved.

As summer approached, we all continued insinuating ourselves into each other's lives—surrogate parents to each other's children, surrogate companions to each other's spouses.

The morning we were caravanning up to Lummi, I was beside myself as to how I might cheer Jake up. After driving for 20 minutes of our two-hour drive, I spontaneously suggested we pull over and swap traveling partners for the rest of the drive. I thought maybe Shari could cheer him up, and whispered that to her as we swapped cars.

Later, that delicious moment under the willow tree with Shari seemed like such a nice break. It had a childlike, innocent quality to it: two kids feeling the beauty of the moment, reaching out to share more of themselves. I felt joy and belonging and, for that moment, I was perfectly in tune with the world. But mostly I felt happy to have a friend like Shari. It seemed like maybe we could all help each other.

When we returned from our long hike, the children were napping inside the cottage. We had set up a tent in the yard to hold excess sleepers and to provide a private space for a couple.

Jake and I planned to sleep in it one night; Greg and Shari the other. In the warm afternoon after our long walk back, Shari and I climbed into the tent to read a bit. By and by, Shari stripped naked.

She turned to me. "We could fool around," she whispered.

My heart pitter-pattered.

"No," I said after a bit, "that wouldn't be fair to Jake. I couldn't do that." My words hung awkwardly in the air and the moment quickly passed.

Later that weekend, the four grown-ups were having a bonfire down at the beach. The kids were asleep in the house. It should have been fun, but Shari and Greg got into a huge fight. Greg stormed off up the stairs.

After a bit of strained silence, I said, "I'll go up and talk to him." I left Shari and Jake by the fire and headed up the long flight of stairs from the beach.

* * *

A week or so later, the girls were back in my kitchen. We wanted to paint hot chili peppers around the salsa cupboard and a grapevine on the other wall. We had just taken the old wallpaper off and were getting ready to clean up for the night. I had stepped out onto the deck, when I heard Jake come home. I glanced inside and saw Shari grab a paintbrush and scrawl the words "I WANT YOU" on the wall, before quickly painting over it. I was momentarily taken aback, a sinking feeling in my gut. Was that a message for me, or for Jake?

Sometime a bit later, we had planned a dinner party for the weekend as usual, but instead of all cooking together, Shari and Jake declared that they were cooking paella for the rest of us. When I tried to help, I was told all the arrangements had been made. Apparently, the two of them had been talking on the phone and come up with a plan. They had arranged to get the ingredients. The night of the paella fest, Shari and Jake were laughing and whispering in the kitchen and I began to get seriously jealous.

Later in the night, I couldn't find Jake and went outside to track him down. Just as I made my way outside, Shari came from around the side of the house and brushed by me. Jake was right behind her.

"Whatcha doing?" I asked, feeling a deep ping of jealousy.

"Just helping Jake get firewood," she responded, but she looked guilty. "Hey, have you seen Greg?" she added too quickly.

"He's inside playing with the kids," I told her, and she left in a hurry.

The incident did not sit well with me. A few days later, I tried to talk to her more directly.

"Shari, what is going on? Is something going on?"

"What do you mean?"

"I'm beginning to feel jealous of you and Jake," I said without mincing words.

"Nothin's going on," she said, then looked at me directly and added with conviction, "Mariah, I will not hurt you."

During this time, I had become active again with my writing and my travel and other personal essays, which were being picked up by magazines regularly. I was also working hard getting ready for the Pacific Northwest Writer's Conference, which was coming up at the end of July. I had earned a spot on the board and was in charge of the Special Event—an evening of festivities where participants and speakers could mingle. The night before the event, Greg was working late and Shari invited us over to her house for dinner. Shari, braless under her tank top, was flirting, obviously vying for Jake's attention, and got pouty when he gave it to me. I was angry and confused as to how to act and feel. Was she pursuing Jake?

The next morning, Jake offered to drop me off at the conference, as some other friends, the Roberts, were caring for

28

the kids. Being stuck there for the day should have been no problem, but somehow it felt wrong. I tried to ignore that gut feeling and busied myself checking in with the other organizers, then headed for a presentation by Jim Molnar of the *Seattle Times*, who had been mentoring me for several months. I should have been interested; instead my underlying unease grew and all of a sudden I felt compelled to go home immediately. Borrowing a vehicle, I left the conference and drove straight home.

I jumped from the truck, dashed through the garage up into the house. As I ran upstairs toward our master bedroom, Jake appeared in the hallway, naked and hard. Behind him in the bedroom was Shari, struggling to pull up her skirt and button up a vest over her exposed breasts.

My eyes locked on hers.

"It's not what you think—" Shari started to say.

"It's not, Shari? It's not! Then what are you doing here with your clothes off?"

"We were having tea . . . and—"

"Don't say that, Shari. It's not true." Jake shook his head.

It was all too obvious. I spun around and pummeled Jake with my fists.

"How could you? I thought you loved me. I thought you both did."

I fell to the floor and sobbed into my hands. I had just witnessed my worst fears come to life, but on some level I couldn't believe it had happened.

Shari and Jake were together—without me? They had an affair—in secret? They left me out? What? How could that be? I thought they loved me?

I couldn't make sense of their deception. Yes, I knew the sexual energy had been running high, but I thought we were all in this together—working out where to go and how to act together. As angry as I was in that moment, even more than that, I felt utterly forsaken—abandoned and alone. My world was crumbling, disintegrating under my feet. Shari and Jake hovered over me as though they weren't sure what to do.

Even as I sat there crying and even under these horrible circumstances, inexplicably, I felt their love and concern. It couldn't be that these two people didn't care about me. At least that is what I desperately needed to believe in that moment—that their love for me was real. And in that moment, in that small gap, grasping for something—anything—to hang on to, I thought, *What if I don't have to be left out?*

Shari had flirted with me in the past, propositioned me, even. Yes, that's it. They left me out because I hadn't been open. While I had said no to her, they had said yes to each other.

In that moment, as an idea formed, I didn't think about where it would lead, how I would feel in the coming days, or how any of this might affect Shari's husband, Greg. All I knew was that I needed the comfort of my two best friends.

"Wait, wait a minute," I said, looking up through tears at them—the two most important people in my life. I was damned if I was going to give up that easily. "Maybe," I said tentatively, "maybe we can take up where you left off."

I stood up and walked toward the bedroom. They followed. We climbed up on the bed. In truth, a part of me was inherently curious, willing to try different things. I imagined this could be simple, playful, and light-hearted—even if it was outside my previous comfort level.

For a beautiful long moment we held each other, finding solace, then we began to explore each other's bodies.

In the end, while the three-way was momentarily comforting, it was not a long-standing solution. Still, the affair had exposed a lot and left me wondering, How did this happen? Why wasn't I enough? What was missing?

Chapter 4

Ashes Are Burning

Sadness is flat and wet, a moldy towel, a flat seven-up, unsweetened chocolate, ash . . . or sadness can feel as full and passionate as an overripe peach, heavy like a brown banana.
~ Journal entry, September 1995

After Shari went home and before falling asleep that night, Jake whispered in my ear almost too quietly to hear, "Please forgive me . . . "

I woke the next morning raw with emotion. I felt like I had no footing to stand on. What had just happened? What had they done? What had I done?

While the previous night's encounter had had a certain sweetness and even exciting hotness to it (it is a classic fantasy, after all), my underlying emotions were complicated. I felt no shame or embarrassment at having been in a three-way, nor did I feel any lingering desire or lust for a repeat performance; ultimately, it did not feel like a sustainable solution.

To make matters worse, I had to return again to the writer's conference. Neither Shari nor Jake could come and I had to go alone. I didn't want to leave. I didn't want to be alone. I didn't want them to be together. Once there, I found myself sitting next to a young man at the coffee bar. I must have looked awful because he asked if I was okay. Before I knew it, I gushed out my whole story to this perfect stranger, hearing the words out of my mouth as if I were someone else telling a tormented love story. Was this my story now?

Somehow I made it through that torturous last day of the conference. Almost immediately afterwards, I resigned from the Pacific Northwest Writer's Board and stopped writing, except in my journals. I suddenly had nothing to say to others. I felt on a gut level that I needed to live the raw experience of my life for some time before I could conceive of writing for publication about it.

In the weeks that followed, it was super-confusing to know how to proceed. Our kids were all still best friends and they wouldn't understand if we suddenly stopped seeing each other, Jake, Shari, and I reasoned together. Plus Shari was terrified that Greg would find out. The three of us decided together that we would act as if nothing had happened and continue to allow our families to get together as usual.

At first this seemed plausible, as I now felt included in the collusion. I thought it would all be okay. I thought I was strong enough to handle it and continue on as if everything was fine.

I had plenty of opportunity to try. Not too long after, it was Shari and Greg's youngest daughter's birthday. We were invited to their house for an outdoor backyard party. In the week before the event, Jake decided that he was going to build a picnic table for them—knowing they were too poor to afford one. It tweaked my insides, but I played along, acting perfectly normal as if it didn't bother me—like I was above anything as petty as feeling upset.

The day of the event, we gamely gathered and everyone ooohed and aahed over the new picnic table. I felt my world getting smaller, and a surreal feeling began to overcome me. On the outside, I was laughing and shooting water pistols with everyone else, but on the inside I was running, screaming, insanely jealous. I held it together that night, but the jealousy was insidious.

I kept wondering what was going to happen to Jake and me, how we were going to rebuild our connection. I poured my heart out into my journals, trying to get the sadness out of my system, so that I could return to normal living. And I would play our special music, hoping to remind him of our closeness. One song, "Ashes Are Burning," by a progressive rock band called Renaissance, echoed my hopes and feelings of this time. I would turn on this music that Jake and I had loved and be overcome by its haunting beauty and meaningful lyrics, and pray that Jake could feel it and remember.

But still, I was jealous and it began affecting my behavior. One day, I drove up to Shari's house and snuck in, knowing she was away. I wanted to look at her phone records. I wanted to know if she and Jake were still talking secretly behind my back. In the dark of her little kitchen, acting as if I was a CIA spy, with the junk drawer open and bills spilled out before me, I couldn't actually focus on the phone records. I felt deeply ashamed. But as the weeks continued, I found I couldn't keep my feelings of hurt and betrayal from overwhelming me.

Now when we all got together, I would often simply lose it. Something would trigger me and a strange dreamlike feeling would grow—the walls would close in on me as they did at the birthday party and my heart would beat wildly. It would end in an overt panic attack, leaving me trembling and crying. The rest of the group, Kate and Phillip Roberts and Greg, had no idea what was wrong with me. Normally cheerful and in control, I was obviously falling apart—seemingly out of the blue. I began to act recklessly too, drinking way too much and doing dangerous things.

One afternoon we had all gathered on our deck for a party. I was already drinking carelessly, when something triggered me. Earlier in the day, Jake had set up a large ladder to trim the huge trees on our side yard. These trees were tall—probably 50 feet tall—and he needed to reach the upper branches. He had come up with the idea that if he used the second-story deck as a base, then his 30-foot ladder could extend up closer to the top of the trees. The ladder was still set up, suspended 40 feet above the ground. In the middle of my anxiety attack, I suddenly went over to it and began frenetically climbing it. When I got close to the top, I turned around and started dancing, showing off for the group.

Everyone called out to me to get down, but I didn't feel like it. Eventually, Jake managed to talk me safely down.

Shortly after this event, Shari became unhinged as well. She feared my erratic behavior was going to draw attention to the affair. One day, she came over and screamed at me.

"You are on a one-woman course of revenge, out to destroy me!" she yelled.

"What are you talking about?" I countered. "You were the one who made the choice that led to these consequences. You. You, who so righteously talk to your kids about cause and effect. You, who prides herself on parenting with natural consequences. You. You were the one who had an affair with my husband, then asked me to watch your kids! Well, guess what? You fucked up big time, girl, and your actions are going to have some natural and difficult consequences."

"You don't know what you are doing," she screamed back. "You're playing with fire."

"What fire, Shari? What? I bet Jake told you about his dream, right? You probably think you're the woman from his dream, don't you?"

At that moment I wanted to punch her and rip her hair out. I wanted to claw at her breast and scream in her face.

She looked at me coldly and said, "I know things Jake will never tell you . . . "

* * *

Rrrring. Rrring.

The sound of the phone trilling after midnight woke me with a start.

"Hello?" I mumbled.

"He's going to kill him!" Shari cried into the phone.

"What? What are you talking about?" I said. "Who is going to kill whom?"

"Greg," she said urgently, breathlessly. "He knows, and he left the house—tires squealing—saying he was going to kill Jake. Mariah, he looked crazy!"

My heart leapt to my throat, pounding wildly. Jake, awake now, looked at me eyebrows raised.

"Jake has to leave the house. Now! He'll be there any minute. He has to leave!" Shari was adamant.

"It's Shari," I mouthed to Jake. "She says she just told Greg and he is on his way over here . . . Shari says he is really mad and we should leave . . . " I told him quietly.

Jake pulled the phone out of my hand.

"I am not going to leave, Shari," he said quietly. "I am going to face him and talk to him. It's okay, don't worry."

"But, Jake, he is really mad, and he is a big guy. I don't think you've ever seen him mad," she protested. "I don't think he is up for a chat . . . "

"I have to go now, Shari," Jake said and hung up.

We lay in bed for a moment. I was trembling and scared.

"We should get up," I said, "get ready."

I had just pulled on my robe when we heard a car pull up to the driveway. I ran downstairs to the front door first and opened it part way. Greg was rushing up the steps, red-faced, holding a pitchfork.

I stood in the entryway, barring his way. Jake was somewhere behind me. Inexplicably, I felt calm and centered. There was no way I was letting him into my house with that weapon.

"Get out of the way, Mariah!" he growled at me. "This is between me and Jake—nothing to do with you."

I looked Greg squarely in the eyes. We were friends, after all. "I am not moving, Greg, until you put down your weapon. You can't enter this house with that weapon."

"Jake! Get out here!" Greg screamed past me wild-eyed.

"Move!" he yelled at me.

"No," I said firmly. "Put down your weapon."

Greg grunted and then put the pitchfork off to the side and made for the front door. I moved to the side quickly as he pushed the door the rest of the way open. Jake was right behind me, and within milliseconds Greg had shoved Jake hard and pushed him against the wall where my antique clock hung. He began strangling Jake with his forearm pushed against his neck.

"Let's take this outside," Greg said.

"Greg, I don't want to fight you. I am so sorry. I am so sorry," Jake repeated over and over again. "I don't want to fight you. You have every right to be angry. I am sorry. I did appreciate our friendship. I am sorry."

Greg screamed that he had thought about coming over and setting fire to our house—something neither of us had thought of. I cried the whole time.

Greg roughed Jake up a little more, punching his shoulder a bit, but soon calmed down. Our young children were upstairs still sleeping and I am sure he considered that. Greg turned on his heel and abruptly left the house, leaving Jake and me standing in the entryway, speechless.

It was over almost as fast as it started. As the adrenaline rush waned, my body, which had been registering fear in the pit of my stomach all day prior to this event, now, strangely, felt nothing. We climbed the stairs silently, and crawled back into bed.

"Are you okay?" I asked Jake.

"Yeah."

In the dark, I tried to imagine a way out of this mess . . . some path back to good times, but I could see only darkness ahead.

"What are we going to do, Jake?" I whispered into the night.

But there was no response . . .

A numbness crept in that by morning would turn into full-blown depression. What an ugly mess we had gotten ourselves into.

Chapter 5

Ask Me Anything

I sat on the therapist's couch, shaking. He had had an affair
with my best friend. It seemed impossible yet true. At some
core part of my being, I felt this was not a death sentence to
our marriage, our love, but just a challenge. The therapist
wanted to know if I wanted to separate. I was shocked at her
question. Of course not, I replied. It's not like that. But
nothing could have prepared me for how close we came to
doing that. I loved him. I loved him in all the ordinary ways,
with jealousy and attachment, with equal parts of hate and
love sometimes. But I loved him in some other even more
fundamental way too. Like how a stream loves its banks, how
the shore loves the waves. I felt everything as my own failing
at unconditional love. I did love him, so how come I was
sitting here? I was not enough? Love is not enough? I
struggled with these concepts.
~ Journal entry, fall 1995

Jake and I decided we had to stop seeing Shari. I had thought
I could handle it, that we could all stay friends, but I couldn't,
and now that Greg knew, it clearly required a parting of the
ways.

As for healing our own relationship, Jake had hoped we could
just get over it all quickly and peacefully. Unfortunately, with my
irrational outbursts and anxiety attacks, we were going to need
help.

I struggled with the idea that our current problem was my

fault. This seemed to have been totally driven by him, right? I mean up to that point we had been happy—just one year earlier for our tenth anniversary, he had redeclared his love and tattooed my name on his ass, for criminey sake. I asked Jake about it and he agreed with me.

"Yes," he said. "We have been happy and close and intimate 90 percent of the time, but the other 10 percent . . . "

I knew what he was referring to. I had terrible PMS (premenstrual syndrome) that would trigger severe mood swings and a dark cloud of depression for several days each month. We would get into fights. I used to joke that it was like clockwork: once a month Jake was an asshole . . .

At the time, I knew that PMS was caused by hormonal shifts, but I didn't realize there were other contributing factors, such as repressed memories and post-traumatic stress, that could exacerbate my symptoms and make me terribly unpredictable and difficult to live with. I also did not believe it was within my power to change.

When we entered couples therapy, our therapist began to point me to the fact that, even though he was the one to have strayed, I might consider that this was an opportunity to work on myself as well. Strangely, this put us on equal footing, and it began to feel like we were embarking on an endeavor together.

We acknowledged we wanted more out of our relationship and more out of life. By chance our therapist, Shanti, with whom we both felt comfortable, was a disciple of Amachi, an Indian woman affectionately known as "the hugging saint." Shanti introduced us to Eastern spiritual books and concepts we had never heard of, having grown up in white suburban America, and we became curious to learn more. Some months into therapy and because of Jake's dream, we began to think about pursuing a more active spiritual path as a means for healing and growing. But what was the doorway in?

One thing that inadvertently lit the way was the night Jake decided to tell me the whole story of his affair. Coincidentally — or maybe not — it was Shari's birthday. I remember in vivid detail sitting in the car that night. We were on our way out to dinner by ourselves and it was raining. I asked him a question, possibly about the affair, and he pulled the car over and stopped on the side of the road.

He turned to me and said, "I have to tell you something."

My heart flip-flopped. I waited. The air was electric.

"It was more than a one-night stand," he said. "It started a couple of months ago, the weekend we all went up to Lummi together, the day after we hiked up the mountain . . . "

And then he proceeded to tell me the whole story, how Shari had placed her hand over his in the car on the way up; how she had come on to him that weekend — actually reaching her hand down his shorts — when the two of them were alone down at the beach bonfire, while I went up to try to calm Greg down after he and Shari had fought. He told me they had met at her house the next day and met another time at a hotel and a couple of other times too, when I discovered them.

"Mariah," he said. "You can ask me anything you want. I will tell you the truth in as much detail as you want."

I couldn't help but remember Shari's words that she knew things Jake would never tell me, and mentioned that to Jake. He said he didn't know what she meant, and that nothing in particular or sinister came to mind. Then he reiterated that he wanted to be transparent and that he would not withhold anything, if that is what I wanted. Later, whenever I requested, we did talk through grisly details. The slate was not pretty, but at least it was clean.

Sitting there in the car on that rainy night, listening to Jake tell me things I didn't want to hear, offering to answer any questions, had a strange effect on me. I felt closer to him in those moments of his sharing than I could have ever imagined. I saw his courage.

I felt honored that he would tell me the truth, however painful it was. It felt like an opening back to intimacy, but we weren't sure where to go next.

Chapter 6

Art of Sexual Ecstasy

Have you ever wished to be touched at the core of your being,
yet felt afraid to open yourself up and be vulnerable?
~ Margot Anand

As Jake and I struggled in that dark fall of our
relationship, when our foundation was shaky and
crumbling, we found ourselves at a crossroads: we
could simply try to go on as usual, burying the pain, letting time
work its magic, or we could use this as an opportunity to dive
deeper into each other, into ourselves, into Life.

At the time, neither of us was remotely religious or spiritual.
Jake was an atheist and I, at best, agnostic. We saw only
hypocrisy in the easily accessible, organized religions of Western
culture. Jake, however, had spent some time when he was
younger reading Carlos Castaneda (an anthropologist who wrote
a series of books about his apprenticeship with a Yaqui Indian
shaman) and was somewhat familiar with Castaneda's concept of
waking up to a different reality. After his Goddess dream Jake
had become interested in the idea of pursuing "enlightenment"—of waking up, he called it, and he underscored that
the Goddess dream had been a startling wake-up call for him.
The trouble was he had no guidelines, and I—well, I didn't even
know what enlightenment was all about, but it sounded better
than the "endarkenment" I was currently experiencing! What
was clear to both of us was that we were in crisis, and that we
had no religious beliefs or balms to fall back on. We needed

something to center us and to point us in a positive direction.

During therapy, we had learned a bit about meditation and were intrigued. Learning to meditate sounded like a good start for a spiritual path. We began perusing the *New Times*, a Seattle periodical dedicated to providing its readers with information and resources on spirituality and personal growth, and learned that the Stonehouse Bookstore in Redmond, Washington, would be hosting a beginning meditation class on Tuesday evenings.

We loved the independent and fanciful Stonehouse Bookstore, aptly named for the craftsman-style historic building that had been made entirely out of local rocks. It looked like something out of a fairytale. We knew the founder was a Swedenborgian pastor, which tickled us because the Wayfarers Chapel where we wed was also Swedenborgian. In choosing the Swedenborgian Wayfarers Chapel to wed, our nonreligious selves appreciated that the founder, Emanuel Swedenborg, had been one of the outstanding scientific figures of his generation in the early 1700s, but spent the end of his life pursuing spiritual questions and insights. Swedenborgian churches today encourage the same spirit of inquiry and personal growth. Just as we had felt comfortable wedding in such a church, we felt comfortable taking a spiritual class sponsored by such an organization.

I remember walking up the steps with a little trepidation that first night, admiring the stones and pretty woodwork, wanting to pause and hunt for a book to lose myself in. The class was in the back, in a small room. There were about eight of us. The teacher talked for 45 minutes about the benefits of meditation, and then said we were going to try it by closing our eyes and counting to ten over and over for five minutes. We were to simply restart counting at one whenever we noticed we had stopped. Five minutes? That seemed an outrageously long time. My mind was racing and active, interested in doing anything but just counting—I wondered what to make for dinner the next night, planned out my outfit for the next day, made up stories about each of the participants, paid attention to sounds in the room—but I did try to follow the directions and would begin counting over when I noticed. After five minutes my legs were tired and twitchy from sitting on the hard floor; it was difficult to imagine meditating for long periods.

Meanwhile, we began to investigate what else was out there. We spent hours perusing the spirituality and New Age sections of bookstores, curious to be introduced to new ideas and ways of thinking. One day I went to the local library and found my way to the self-help section, a section I had never visited before. As I was reaching up to grab a book, another book literally fell off the shelf at my feet, like some sort of spiritual cliché. I picked up *Love Is Letting Go of Fear*, by Gerald G. Jampolsky. I was immediately attracted to it, checked it out, and later read it cover-to-cover. It was the first personal improvement book I had ever read, and its theme became significant to me on my journey.

Somewhere along the way—because hot steamy nights had always been important to us—we picked up a book called *The Art of Sexual Ecstasy: The Path of Sacred Sexuality for Western Lovers*, by Margot Anand. In the book, she referred to practices she called "Tantric," based on an ancient Eastern science that includes sexuality as a doorway to ecstasy and enlightenment. We were delighted with the possibility of a path that included sexuality as a doorway to enlightenment and also intrigued that the book mentioned the importance of meditation. On page 45, we read:

You may wonder what meditation has to do with sensuality and lovemaking. In a nutshell, it provides clarity. Imagine a bottle filled with sand and water. Shake it, and you can't distinguish a thing. This is the way the human mind functions during most of our normal, daily, waking life. It is processing so many thoughts, perceptions and pieces of information that [it] is continuously "blurred." Often the circuits are jammed.

But if you set the bottle down and leave it for a few minutes, the sand will arrange itself in a harmonious layer on the bottom, and the water will become clear. In a way, meditation does the same . . . In long-term relationships there is a tendency for lovemaking to become routine, an automatic process, and this reduces the couple's capacity for enjoyment. By quieting the mind, meditation allows freshness and innocence to return to the act of lovemaking. In fact, meditation in High Sex can be seen as a process of deautomating sexuality.

As much promise as the book seemed to have, however, it sat on our shelf untouched after our initial review. We sometimes scanned it for pictures, hoping for a quick fix—maybe a new position that would enliven us—but, other than that, we had a hard time diving into it. The terms she used were unfamiliar and overwhelming.

One day I picked up a copy of *New Times* and there was a full-length article entitled "Sex and Spirituality—An Interview with Margot Anand." I recognized the name, of course, because of her book. I pored over the article, where Margot Anand described sex as a door to the divine and Tantra as a mystical path. *I want to go on a mystical path*, I thought.

I kept reading, enthralled. Margot went on to say that by practicing SkyDancing Tantra the heart would open to trust, and the mind would learn the art of visualizing, focusing, meditating, and letting go. We could sure use that!

I was intrigued until the article started talking about one partner versus several partners on the path. My stomach knotted at the thought of Jake with other partners . . . *This path sounds risky. Is it just a cover-up for a big free-love orgy? Not my thing.*

But then, she topped off her interview with the enticing proclamation that you would realize your partner is a god or goddess—a magical being—with infinite potentialities in manifestation, able to create their lives as they wish to see them created. *That's what I want!*

At the end of the article was a small notice that Margot Anand herself was going to be in town to give a public lecture at Seattle University Church on Friday in a couple of weeks and that she would be leading a workshop on Tantra the following two days.

I sat there holding the article, debating the possibility of going to that weekend workshop. I wasn't entirely sure I wanted to even show it to Jake. On the one hand, the potential was palpable: Perhaps our sex life, which had positively fueled us before, could be harnessed for something greater? *Perhaps sex is a doorway to the unknowable for us, a doorway to spirituality—a doorway to more?* one part of my brain argued.

You are considering learning about sex in a group setting? the other side screamed. *Are you crazy? Sex is private. I don't want to air our sex life in a group setting. Besides, do you really want to expose each other to a whole bunch of potential sex partners now?*

But, as loud as my fear thoughts were, I knew we had to do something—even if it was risky. Sex, while currently at the heart of our rift, had also been the source of much happiness and play. It seemed like it could be a springboard for us to explore more, to reconnect. We could learn from a Master.

I decided to show the article to Jake.

"What do you think?" I asked nervously, not entirely sure what answer I wanted to hear.

He had no initial qualms. "Wow! This is great. Yes. This is what I want," he said. "I think we should go!"

We signed up and paid for the upcoming workshop (paying in advance was significant, it turned out) and booked a room at the Green Tortoise Hostel nearby. The first session was an informational evening at Seattle University Church, available to the public the night before the workshop was to commence.

As we approached the door that first evening, Jake got an intense case of the willies. He tended to be shy in new social scenes and this was a whopping new scene.

"This is a really stupid idea," he said. "I don't want to do this . . . There is no way I am going through those doors . . . Let's go. Let's leave."

"Um, okay," I responded. "I guess we can try and get our money back from the organizers and the hostel."

There was a long pause as Jake considered which was more embarrassing and painful: asking for our money back . . . losing our money . . . or taking a risk and trying it out.

"Well, I guess we are here. Let's just go hear what she has to say. We can always change our minds and not attend the rest of the workshop." Jake was not one to give up and hated to ask for his money back.

That weekend workshop opened our eyes in ways we couldn't have imagined. We started by learning about soul gazing, a simple technique where you and your partner gaze deeply into each other's eyes for a few minutes—focusing on one eye. In our normal day, we don't do this. We flit our attention in and out, multi-tasking, avoiding too much direct eye contact because it feels invasive. When you do so intentionally, it is like inviting someone into your most private space. It is scary, because the other person can likely see any hidden emotions, desires, or fears reflected in your eyes, and it can be hard to keep emotions from rising inside you. Thus, it requires a certain amount of vulnerability. When we did this at the workshop—in the middle of our mess—it was essentially a reciprocated invitation to be present with each other—not escaping, not hiding or averting, not blaming. Just sitting, looking deeply into each other. Maybe, just maybe, we were after the same thing after all.

During that weekend workshop, we also experienced a bit of what it was like to talk and share in a group setting. It wasn't as intimidating as I thought it would be, and it was interesting to hear what other people had to share. By Saturday night, we felt a whisper of possibility that more was available to us—broken as we were: more in our sex life, more in our relationship, more from life.

Just before lunch on the second day, Margot handed out a flyer announcing an integral part of her SkyDancing Tantra Institute: a yearlong "Love and Ecstasy Training," which was to commence in February in California. The structure of the training, which spanned a 12-month period, was three ten-day sessions in which the participants met as a group to learn various practices designed to increase intimacy, heal sexuality, and bring joy to their lives. For the months in between, participants were encouraged to form smaller regional groups that met one weekend a month to practice. We were advised that Margot's training courses filled up quickly, so you had to commit early if you wanted to go. Plus, if you were complete newbies, as we were, there was an additional prerequisite four-day course prior to the main training. The next prerequisite course was scheduled to begin in less than a month, in November in Malibu, California.

At lunch we went out to a restaurant across the street, fingering the flyer and fairly bursting with possibility. What had seemed overwhelming, only two days before, now was alluring and intriguing. The tiny weekend taste made us hungry.

The debate about what we should do with our lives and with each other came down to this moment in the restaurant. Deciding to take Margot Anand's yearlong training would propel us down a strange and terribly vulnerable path. It would take us out of our comfort zone.

"Do you think we could . . .?" we whispered.

"Would you want to?"

"Should we consider it?"

"What about the kids?"

"How would we work out that much time off from our jobs?"

Here we were at the most exposed and tentative point in our relationship to date, just four months after the affair, at a time when we might have been finger pointing and blaming, at a time when we might have buried our heads in the sand, or separated, and instead we were discussing diving into something new and exciting *together*, something, we suspected, that would challenge us to our core. Of course I worried.

Sex Training? Is this going to be like some crazy commune? Sounds risky—how will we keep our marriage intact? What if I am overcome with jealousy and make a scene? What vulnerabilities might get exposed? Will this bring us closer or drive us apart? What kind of mother am I, thinking of leaving my little kids?

Still, sitting there, contemplating this outrageous venture, I felt curious. This was a journey, I realized, where we would be traveling to an unknown destination on a marital raft about as reliable and safe as the driftwood and kelp raft that launched our relationship so many years before. But one thing Jake and I had always done well was traveling. We used to say, if you really want to see if you can get along with someone, go backpacking through Europe for two months together, or go sailing for a month. We had done both and many other crazy adventures. But this, this inner journey we were contemplating, were we prepared for this? In the end, it sounded like a grand adventure and we were willing to try. The joint decision made me hope that despite the recent events, our love for each other and for our own selves was, on some deeper level, stronger than the tenuous threads of our current broken storyline.

Yet it seemed an impossible endeavor logistically: three ten-day sessions, plus one weekend every month for a year? How on earth would we pull that off? But from one moment to the next, we looked past all the logistics, connected with each other, and said, "Let's do it!"

Before we had time to change our minds, we had committed to the yearlong love and ecstasy training in Northern California and the prerequisite four-day workshop in Malibu.

This decision threw us completely out of sync with our normal, suburban, parenting lives and goals, and gave us a focus that had nothing to do with engineering, paralegal work, diapers, or school. We began to devour Margot Anand's book. What is sacred space? What is the inner flute? What is Kundalini? What is a chakra? What is the Wave of Bliss? It was scary, exciting, and fun.

We had worried about the kids and our jobs, but when we announced to our parents that we wanted to do this, they quickly offered up live-in babysitting service. As for our jobs, we took the forthright approach and simply advised our supervisors that we would be away for these three ten-day periods next year, taking leave without pay for any time over our entitled vacation time.

Thankfully, we had no idea of what was to come . . . but my dream that night seemed to hint that the way might be challenging:

I walked downstairs and saw that in the middle of the living room a mountain had appeared from nowhere.

"Jake!" I called. "Look!"

He came downstairs and stood next to me. We looked from each other to the mountain now standing in the middle of our living room—the top disappearing through what once had been our ceiling. It was impossibly steep and high, with treacherous crevasses and lots of snow.

"There's a mountain in our living room," I said, giving voice to the obvious. "What should we do, Jake?"

"Climb it, of course—together!" was his dream-self's reply.

I woke feeling that a dangerous journey was imminent, yet simultaneously feeling the pixie in me emerge. She was excited to climb that living-room mountain, just like she had been when she pushed the rickety raft away from the safety of shore that summer long ago, unsure if she would float long enough to make it to a distant safe shore, but willing to try.

This journey I'm on is a journey to freedom—to a place on the cliff's edge. I've been at the cliff's edge physically before. It's an amazing feeling. Now to get there emotionally. This is an adventure of the mind, of consciousness. Yes, you could fall climbing, but without trying, you risk never feeling the intensity. I am climbing the cliffs of consciousness.

(Journal entry, 8 November 1995)

The night before we headed off to the first week of love and ecstasy training, I had another dream. In it, I died. I didn't know that you could dream that you died. I had heard if you did dream such a thing, then you would actually die. But I didn't. In the dream I was floating with Jake above a scene happening below.

Jake turned to me and said, "Look! Someone has drowned." He pointed to a bunch of family members who were walking in the surf below and had just come upon a body. "I think it's you."

My dream-self looked down just as his dad pulled a body up out of the seaweed. It was mine. I could even see that I was wearing a white tank top.

All of a sudden, the shock was too great, and I woke from the dream screaming and crying. To look down and see your own dead body is amazing. Once awake, I reflected that my dream seemed to symbolize to me that a big change or the end of some part of my life was coming, because I was still so alive watching it all.

We arrived at the resort later the next day. As scary as it was to go to this wild, other side of life—this "Love and Ecstasy" group retreat—we felt comfortable and safe. The retreat was well structured, and the leader, Margot Anand, was a trained psychologist. We learned you were allowed to participate either as "deep divers," sticking primarily with one partner as Jake and I were doing (which helped me relax), or as a "free floater" moving from partner to partner for various exercises. There was to be no explicit sexual exchange during the training sessions. Everything was deliberate and planned—a necessity, perhaps, when 40 people from around the country gather to delve into sexual ecstasy techniques together.

The setting in Napa Valley was gorgeous. The retreat took place at White Sulphur Springs Resort & Spa in St Helena, California, which we found to be quite charming, with quaint rooms and cottages situated on 44 acres in a canyon. There were hiking trails over creeks and near waterfalls through redwoods, madrones, and Douglas fir trees, not to mention abundant poison oak (which got me into trouble at one spontaneous outdoor session with Jake on a hike in the woods . . . turns out, I am incredibly sensitive to poison oak).

The resort itself had its own sulphur spring, and there were outdoor soaking pools open 24 hours, plus you could sign up for mud baths or massages, if you wanted. There was a large meeting room at the lodge sufficient for all 40 participants to comfortably meet and learn together; we gathered there three times per day. A wonderful crew, who made healthful and super-yummy vegetarian food, catered the event.

One of the caterers was this flamboyant woman who came dressed up every day in a costume with wings, flowing skirts, and sparkly shoes. She was missing a front tooth. I talked to her one day. She told me she was the Tooth Fairy. I laughed, but she persisted. "No, really, I am!" Then she went to her purse and pulled out her wallet, and there was the proof, her official California state driver's license, which identified her as "Tooth Fairy." I laughed and told her I couldn't wait to get home to my three- and six-year-old kids to let them know I had actually met the Tooth Fairy while away!

We gathered the first evening for an introductory talk in the big meeting room, where we were instructed to set our intentions for the retreat. I wrote in my journal that my intentions were to awaken my Kundalini—something I knew nothing about, but that intrigued me—to give my partner space, and to learn the vulnerable side of intimacy. During that first gathering, I watched, mesmerized, as a caterpillar slowly crossed the entire length of the big room as we all talked and set our intentions. I thought to myself that we were all caterpillars on our way, hopefully, to becoming butterflies. Transformation was afoot.

Chapter 7

Kundalini Rising

Knowledge is certain; the search for personal knowing is very, very hazardous. Nobody can guarantee it. If you ask me if I can guarantee anything, I say I cannot guarantee you anything. I can only guarantee danger; that much is certain. I can only guarantee you a long adventure with every possibility of going astray and never reaching the goal . . . But one thing is certain: the very search will help you to grow. I can guarantee only growth. Danger will be there, sacrifice will be there; you will be moving every day into the unknown, into the uncharted, and there will be no map to follow, no guide to follow . . . to accept the challenge of the unknown is the only way to grow.

~ Osho

On day three of the first session of love and ecstasy training, in a circle of 40 people, Jake and I were in the middle of an exercise called "dynamic streaming," the goal of which was to awaken our Kundalini, or as Margot paraphrased it, your "ecstatic response." Kundalini, I had learned over the course of the last several months, is a kind of energy or force that typically lies dormant at the base of the spine, like a coiled serpent. When awakened, this energy apparently runs unchallenged up the spine and can stimulate a profound mystical experience. However, we were also warned that it is a very powerful energy and that it is dangerous to work with it outside of a controlled environment. Kundalini has been described as a kind of highly creative intelligence that dwarfs our own intelligence and requires surrender. We learned that there was such a thing as a Kundalini crisis or Kundalini syndrome in which the symptoms resembled those of a Kundalini awakening, but were overwhelming or out of control.

Jake was completely excited about the possibility of awakening Kundalini. He wanted to go for it. He didn't care a whit about any warnings or possible dangers—that was for sissies, he claimed. "More, Now, Faster" was sort of his motto. When we started taking a Kundalini yoga class for couples in Seattle around this time, always looking for more Kundalini, we learned a "Venus Kriya," an exercise that included soul gazing with your palms touching your partner's palms, and fire breathing together (a kind of short, fast, shallow, forceful breath). We were told the exercise helped combine male and female polarities. We were warned that these were very powerful techniques and should not be done for longer than three minutes at a time. It was said you could actually start sharing the consciousness of your partner, which sounds awesome, but could be dangerous if it happened while driving for instance. Jake was intrigued, and immediately thought we should test the limits.

"Let's do this for an hour," he said. "Let's see what happens!"

I too was a sucker for experiencing more, for getting closer. Generally our approach to all exercises we were taught was to be, at the least, diligent in our pursuit, and usually pushing any recommended limits. We didn't believe there was any real danger. And even as much as we desired something more, we didn't completely believe in the *actual* possibility of experiencing more, such as subtle energies or psychic incidents or anything woo woo, per se.

As novel as the undertaking was for us as a whole, it still came as a surprise when, almost right from the start, I began to have glimpses of new and mystical, seemingly unfathomable experiences. I quickly felt like Dorothy in *The Wizard of Oz*. I had a feeling we were not in Kansas anymore.

One of the first things that happened to me took place during the morning meditation at the first ten-day session. Although we were not experienced meditators and still felt ill-prepared to sit for long stretches, we were still bound and determined to participate in every part of the retreat, so we always went to the morning yoga and meditation. We found it got easier to sit quietly in a large group of people who were also sitting quietly.

By and by I began to have strange visions during these morning meditations. An experienced meditator might have ignored the visions while seeking a more pure experience of an undistracted mind. But I was inexperienced and had never seen a "vision" before, so I really didn't understand what was happening. I was curious about them, but had absolutely no idea what they were or what they meant. One day, during one of the breaks, I decided to describe the strange pictures that came to my mind during meditation to a small group of participants. One girl turned toward me and told me I was describing different Tarot cards. She showed me cards from her set and I was flabbergasted. What? No way. I had never even seen traditional Tarot cards before this. I don't recall all the cards she said I described, but I do recall that one of them was the "Three of Swords," and another was the "Knight of Swords." I was fascinated that my mind could come up with pictures that actually existed, but that I had never seen before. The Knight of Swords (a charging knight on horseback with raised sword) symbolizes charging forward with great momentum and with apparently little regard to the dangers one may encounter. It is a card of fearlessness and invincibility. The Three of Swords (a heart with three swords piercing it amid a terrible storm) is about abandonment, betrayal, and extreme pain, but when it shows up in a reading, it indicates an opportunity to expand and learn, and is likely indicative of the ability to conquer any pain that comes your way.

I began having more visions too. One time I had a hard time

meditating because I kept seeing a mother and child image. I couldn't understand what it might mean to me. I mentioned it to a fellow participant who had been seated near me; she looked at me strangely, then said that at the meditation that morning she had been working on healing her relationship with Christianity and was thinking about Mother Mary and Jesus the whole time. She mused that I might have been picking up on her thoughts. I had no idea such a thing was possible.

Another time I saw very clearly two cupped hands holding a large, upright crystal. I didn't think too much of it, until on the last day, Margot closed the week by holding a large crystal in her two cupped hands in front of the whole group. It was exactly what I had seen earlier in the week. That was a little eerie.

Still nothing got my attention quite as strongly as what happened on the third day during the dynamic streaming exercise. This exercise took place at the middle session of the day. We had already done yoga and meditated and had received some instructions to prepare us for the dynamic streaming practice. The exercise was supposed to help us understand the orgasmic process energetically so that we could feel such energy independent of the sexual process. We were to learn how to relax in high states of arousal and to open the body up to the possibility of a full body orgasm on an energetic level. Essentially, it was supposed to stimulate the Kundalini energy coiled at the base of the spine.

Prior to the start of the exercise, I was already feeling a little off. I couldn't put my finger on it exactly, but I felt tingly all over, expectant maybe. I had gone for a walk through the woods prior to the session, and ended up running wildly because of the pent-up energy I felt. I came to the session with bits and pieces of plants and twigs stuck in my hair and slightly out of breath.

This particular exercise was a partner exercise with one giving and one receiving. We decided I would receive first. I needed to calm down and catch my breath. The exercise involved some relaxation techniques, and then the receiver was to stand up, leaning over slightly, while the giver began vibrating minute sections of the spine from the base on up. Jake began doing the exercise, vibrating up my spine and suddenly—from Jake's perspective—I slumped to the ground and was unresponsive. From my perspective, I found myself in the middle of an overpowering vision. An enormous anaconda-type snake had wrapped itself around my body and was crushing me. The room in which the rest of the 40 participants were still practicing receded from my view, although I was vaguely aware of it. There was some sort of whispering in my ear—the experience was terrifying, but also strangely compelling. I couldn't move physically. Jake was frantically talking to me, but I couldn't respond—didn't even want to respond. I had the feeling that I could disappear into that vision and never return. It felt very dark, yet terribly seductive. I was mesmerized even as I was being crushed.

Meanwhile, Jake was beginning to realize that I was *really* not responding. He got the attention of the teachers without leaving my side. Jake explained to me later that Margot herself came over to me. I could sense her presence, but I was still gripped with the vision of the snake and the compelling urge not to listen to anything else. Margot grabbed my face with both hands and looked me straight in the eyes.

"Come back!" she said, and then, "You *will* come back to this room right now!"

I was not inclined to listen to her. She grabbed my face again, looked me in the eyes, and repeated, "COME BACK NOW!"

I sort of came to and was released from the vision. I was trembling from head to toe and could not stop shaking for hours afterward. Margot instructed Jake and me to sit in the corner of the room. She told Jake to imagine a psychic wall of protection around me and to stand guard. I really didn't understand what was happening. I felt completely spent—like a shell of myself. It took hours to recover. We missed the whole rest of the session. I was glad that Jake was sitting like a sentry near me. Although exhausted and confused, I felt safe and protected.

There was no question: I was not in Kansas anymore.

Chapter 8

Release and Retreat

The pelvis is at the center of our physical structure. It is a large strong receptacle, holding vital organs and major muscles of locomotion. But it also holds some of our strongest feelings and attitudes.

~ Jack Painter

Jake and I had entered into the love and ecstasy training because we wanted to experience more intimacy, more ecstasy, more connection, and more spirituality. Many of the participants, however, came because they wanted to heal from various incidents. At the time, it never occurred to me that I might need any sort of sexual healing. I felt healthy and was secure in the fact that I had a happy childhood. My parents were loving and kind. Everything was good . . . well, everything was good, except this nagging feeling that there was . . . well, something . . . something that was not quite right. I chocked it up to the infidelity. That was bad enough for me.

What I hadn't considered was that there were secrets hiding in the dark closets of my mind and nether regions. Later, I came to think of these secrets as scorpions, which if left unexposed, lay in wait to sting me when unwittingly provoked. But at the time, I had never looked inside, had never traveled to the basement of my mind, had never investigated why I was afraid of flying, or dying, or why I was afraid of being abandoned. I had never considered that it didn't have to be that way.

We continued on with love and ecstasy training. The culmination of cycle one was something called "pelvic release." Pelvic release is a kind of deep massage of the entire inner and outer pelvic region. On women, the idea is to massage gently and easily both outside and inside the *yoni* (the term Margot Anand used for vagina), even reaching to the cervix, paying attention to any spots that are more sensitive than others. On men, it includes massaging around the perineum, *vajra* (her term for penis) and prostate, accessed through the anus.

We learned that men and women hold tensions in their internal pelvic organs, often due to the build-up of repressed anger against abusers. These tensions prevent the tissues from feeling any sensations, and may keep the person living with perpetual post-traumatic stress syndrome (PTSS). "Often, people even become anorgasmic," Margot described, "and they think it is for life! But it doesn't have to be."

We received specific instructions. Margot told us, "You want to massage the interior tissues of the vagina or anus until the receiver indicates they feel a point of tension or until the giver finds a spot that might feel like a single or several 'hot' nodules of tissue." When a spot is located, we learned, the receiver puts all their awareness on it, while the giver begins applying pressure. As the pain increases, the receiver practices special, deep breathing techniques and works the pelvic muscles while holding eye contact with the giver. The goal is to accept the pain and release it through the breath.

"As the nodule lets go of the tension, intense heat is released and the tissue begins to feel again," Margot coached. "And there is often some emotional release, such as crying, or even screaming, as the process may stimulate traumatic memories," she further explained to reassure us that such a response was normal.

We began to appreciate that this was delicate work, exposing deep vulnerability, and that it needed to be done with respect, with sacred ritual, and with sustained eye contact, so that the receiver felt safe and protected. Margot stressed the importance of ongoing communication during the process. The giver was to gently ask the receiver to share whatever was happening—senses, feelings, thoughts—to keep them from shutting down. We discovered there is a balance that can be achieved between not enough pressure, which results in nothing being evoked, and too much pressure, which results in a kind of armoring taking over. The exercise helps the receiver recognize resistance and struggle, and to move past it, essentially acknowledging its existence and participating in its release.

This kind of release work, sometimes called myofascial release or somatic therapy, is based on the idea that we hold body memories, or "tissue memories." When trauma occurs, whether physical, mental, emotional, or a combination of these, the myofascia, or muscle and connective tissue, hold the memory and are literally the record keeper of the memory in the body/mind complex. In a controlled setting, such as a pelvic release session, one may be able to release the stored negative feelings, so as to heal.

For this part of the retreat we had a visiting lecturer, Jack Painter. Jack was a pioneer in the work of postural integration, which is a body-based therapy that combines deep tissue massage, breath work, and energy flow. Painter prepared a modified introductory training for us in pelvic release. The goal was to learn how to help our partners and ourselves release and integrate feelings and energy blocked in the inner pelvis through three methods: 1) breath work; 2) deep connective tissue work on the muscles of pelvic floor, anus, prostate, and G-spot; and 3) emotional expression and gestalt therapy.

The day Painter came to the retreat and talked to us, Jake was keyed up and excited. Part of Painter's lectures included detailed internal and external pelvic anatomy. He showed us drawings of all the different parts of male and female genitalia, including the muscles and fascia of both the male and female perineum, all the male and female genital organs, as well as details of the penis and vagina. Jake paid close attention to all the details. Painter went on to give explicit directions on how to probe the entry points of the pelvis so that the receiver would relax and allow further exploration. We were in uncharted territory here, intentionally exploring traditionally forbidden areas, like the anus and rectum. He taught us how to hook at the inner, ringed structure of the anus and give outward broadening stretches, while doing charging and discharging breath work. He warned that there might be anger present and to allow it—even stimulate it, if possible. He described the nerve plexus at the base of the sacrum, which helped bring our energy and feelings out in the open. We might explore feelings of shame or wanting to hide when this was stimulated.

The lecture was not sexual so much as clinical at this point. Jake took it all in, like an 11-year-old kid at an exciting school science demonstration, eager to learn and to practice. It seemed a little like overkill to me. I kept thinking, *Do we really have to learn all this stuff? I mean, we know what's down there and how to use it, right?* But on the other hand, I also knew our home practice was going to include doing pelvic release sessions with each other, so I was glad Jake had paid close attention and was totally into it. Despite the subject matter, I began to appreciate the reverence that came with the practice. At all stages along the way, the giver was to maintain eye contact, check in with the receiver, proceed with permission, and explore this territory together intentionally. The practice was based on an underlying commitment to help one another. At the end of any practice session we shared feedback. We asked each other, "What was that like for you? What worked? What was troubling?" We practiced listening without comment to the responses. I began to appreciate the importance of allowing a space for feelings to be fully expressed, whatever they were, and listening to the response. Sometimes the hardest part in life is to allow another person to share their feelings. My default position is to try to control those feelings, or to be afraid of them . . . not my most shining hour. Through this journey, I've come to appreciate that our feelings never go away—we just learn to accept them.

After our detailed lecture on pelvic release we were encouraged to practice on our own. Jake and I returned to our little cottage at the resort and began to prepare our sacred space in preparation for this new practice. At the training we had learned that creating a sacred space for lovemaking was essential. In her book, *The Art of Sexual Ecstasy*, Margot Anand says:

> A sanctuary protects you from the hubbub of the ordinary world. It lifts you up and out of ordinary reality. It possesses distinct qualities that set it apart: silence, beauty, elegance, sensual delight. It engenders feelings of confidence and harmony and sets the stage for moments of special grace, for being your best, for experiences of the highest quality . . . This sanctuary should not only afford protection from the outside world, but positively contribute to extraordinary lovemaking. It should be your Persian garden of pleasure, your Tantric temple of sexual fulfillment, your Japanese teahouse of ultimate delight. This is your Sacred Space, a place designed to create the conditions for ecstatic lovemaking. It is an environment for bliss.

We set up a little altar with a pretty scarf I had brought along and added some tokens, like a pinecone or rock that we had found on our walks, along with photos of our kids. We tied some other silk scarves together and made a circle around the bed to further define our sacred space. We were not allowed to have candles in the room, so instead we hung a string of Christmas lights. These few touches transformed our room and set the stage. We were entering into sacred space. We were protected, safe. We could explore whatever came up. I can say in hindsight it was exceedingly important to enter into the space with intention and protection, as I had no idea what was coming next.

* * *

At the end of the first cycle, we had chosen a smaller group of participants with whom we clicked and formed a regional group that was to meet one weekend per month between sessions. As it turned out, our "regional" group was not actually regional to us. The rest of our group was comprised of Northern Californians, and we would have to travel from Seattle to the San Francisco area to meet up with them. We liked these people, though, and except for the added expense of traveling, we were happy to do so.

These weekend getaways were eye-opening in a whole other way from the retreat. We got a glimpse into the lifestyles of different folks. During these "regional" meetings, we had a chance to stay at many multimillion-dollar dwellings, including a historic mansion owned by a successful businessman right in the heart of San Francisco. Another time, we visited a huge mansion up in the mountains of Marin County, north of San Francisco, that had an Olympic-size swimming pool and gorgeous panoramic views. Two of the participants got engaged while we were there. One time we met in Los Angeles at a beautiful, high-end home that was in the middle of foreclosure. The participant who invited us, named "Lucky," had an unusual business. He squatted in the homes of those who had been evicted and whose homes were about to be foreclosed. The owners asked him to be there, because as soon as there was a squatter on site, the whole eviction process had to start again, gaining the homeowners some three additional months in which to buy their home back out of default. "Lucky" moved from beautiful home to beautiful home without paying a dime.

One of our favorite weekend gatherings was at the home of Kami, who was a quintessential backcountry herb woman. She lived way out in the country near Vacaville, California, in a house that she had built entirely herself from recycled lumber and other materials she had picked up along the way. Her house had cost $9000 to build all-in, and that included her biggest splurge: a $2000 composting toilet. Her charming little 500-square-foot rustic cabin had a wood stove in the living room and shelves upon shelves of herbs in the kitchen. We all camped out together on pads. She had made a back deck of sorts on which sat an old, claw-foot tub, and invited us to take nice, hot soaks right there in nature. The only sounds were those of a nearby babbling brook and the cries of birds of prey on the wind. You could sit outside her primitive simple house, surrounded by big fir trees while soaking in the deep tub, and feel a kind of extravagance all its own. She was a wild woman, who headed into the hills behind her house in a long skirt and bare feet to gather mushrooms and herbs: oat straw, rosemary, sage, burdock, dandelion, purslane, mullein, and so many more, which she ate, or from which she made tinctures and teas. I liked her. She was a down-to-earth free spirit. During the weekend we spent with her, we indulged in awakening our senses in ways heretofore foreign to us. She took us down to the creek near her house and told us the mud had healing qualities. We all stripped nude in the warm summer day, away from the judging eyes of civilized folk, and covered our entire bodies and faces and hair in mud. It was strangely freeing, being covered in mud—as if we were entirely behind a mask. We frolicked like children or wood nymphs on the banks of that creek. Jake, who is normally terribly finicky about sticky things, had a big grin on his face and said "Mariah, you look beautiful!"

Outside the formal training session we were also introduced to Harbin Hot Springs, one of the oldest and most beautiful natural hot springs in California, located above the Napa Valley wine region. Harbin hosts workshops and retreats as well as day visitors. It sits on over 5000 acres of privacy among undeveloped woodland. The springs vary from extremely hot to soothingly warm to breathtakingly cold. Clothing is optional. The setting is quiet and reverent, with people gathering in meditative silence. I learned here that nakedness does not have to mean being exposed and judged so much as protected and accepted.

These informal weekend retreats were important for Jake and me. After the affair, we both lost our best friends and our main social outlet, and we were still tentative with each other. These outings gave us the chance to relax and play together while forming new friendships.

Chapter 9

The Petersons

Mommy, I'm scared of the dark, there's monsters out there.
~ Journal entry, 1996

On our own time, sometimes at the retreats, sometimes during the weekend sessions with our regional groups, and sometimes at home, we began working on the pelvic release exercises. When I was the receiver, Jake would gently begin exploring and deliberately massaging my pelvic region as we had been taught. We worked together, with him asking permission to proceed further and my granting it, as I was ready. The first time he did this was during the initial cycle in the resort room that we had turned into our sacred space. I had worked on Jake and we had switched roles, with him now working on me. The session was going well when he reached the part where he was to press on my G-spot. I told him it felt like something was there, which meant that he was to apply more pressure while we did the breath work that helped the energy discharge. All of a sudden I had a vision of a man's face. I began to talk about it with Jake and later recorded it in my journal. I told him it was a "looming, scary, dark, evil" face. I said it belonged to Don Peterson, the dad of a family we used to be friends with when I was very young. I told Jake, "I don't feel like I can keep myself safe." Then I had another partial flash and described a basement room with a dirt floor, a mattress, and a washer and dryer.

I could not really make any sense out of the partial flash

images, but the feelings were intense. I was shaking all over. I couldn't continue on with the exercise. I was scared. The episode triggered a full-blown anxiety attack, which I would later come to learn was a post-traumatic stress episode.

We didn't really know what to make of this sudden vision and anxiety attack, so we just treated it as a feeling and worked on trying to dissipate the feelings by concentrating on the breath work. Eventually, I was able to calm down, and we decided we had done enough for this session, but we kept on practicing at the retreat and at home, too, and I kept on having flash memories, sometimes of the oldest brother, Larry, too.

Along with these strange, partial flashes of Don and Larry Peterson, I began having dreams as well. I recorded the following in my journal:

> The most amazing set of circumstances has been happening. It's almost too much, too coincidental, too bizarre.
> I started having flash memories of the Petersons:
> - scary face – Don
> - dream about Denise
> - dream about the mom
> - weeping willow tree on land near Preston, WA
> - Larry scared, bad
> - stick story
> (Journal entry, 1996)

This was a very odd time for me. The flashbacks came with powerful anxiety attacks and I couldn't understand where these flashbacks were coming from. Plus the dreams seemed to involve Denise, the youngest of the Petersons, whom I barely remembered. The basement room that had a dirt floor kept showing up in my flash visions. Somehow it seemed connected to the Petersons, but intellectually it didn't make sense to me, because I knew the Petersons lived in a one-story house. Was this a neighbor's house? How was it significant? Why did it keep coming up for me? Why did I keep dreaming about the Petersons? Was I going crazy?

* * *

Over the course of the next few months, and generally connected with love and ecstasy practices, sudden visions or "memories" involving the Peterson family continued to surface. I already had certain easily accessible memories. The Petersons had been friends of our family and lived a couple of blocks away from us, until we moved to a different neighborhood when I was seven. I think we got to know each other because my dad and the Petersons' dad worked together. At any rate, our families gathered with some regularity: we often celebrated Thanksgiving and sometimes Boxing Day (the day after Christmas) together; we went to each other's kids' swim meets and soccer games, and went camping together on occasion. They took care of me when my mom went to the hospital the week before Christmas to have my baby brother. I was three and a half then. I have one indelible memory of that time. I was looking out the living room window, waving goodbye to my mom and dad. A Christmas tree was in the corner. For years I was confused about that memory, because I thought Mom and Dad had left me home alone, and I couldn't understand why they would do that. It turns out, it wasn't our house; it was the Petersons', which had exactly the same layout as our house.

My mom tells me I used to stay at the Petersons' house once a week after school when I was less than five. I don't remember much of the details of that time, except eating Campbell's Scotch Broth soup; it was comforting to me, a touch of home, I think. Later my mom told me it was the only thing I would eat.

At one point our two families purchased a couple of adjacent, 5-acre parcels of wooded land in Preston, Washington. My dad dreamed of building a house out there. He made a model house out of popsicle sticks to show us what it would look like. We used to go up to that land and walk the property. Its wet, earthy scent mixed with the skunk cabbage of those Washington State woods; purple foxgloves and red snapdragons grew wild on the dirt road up to our site. One day, I walked into the woods and looked around and couldn't see any of the grown-ups. I wasn't sure of the way out and appeared to be surrounded by banana slugs— gross! I cried out for help. My dad came and carried me out on his shoulders, but the Peterson dad sneered at me and called me a baby.

The part I liked best about visiting that land in the woods was a mature weeping willow tree on land nearby. I wished it were on our property. The branches reached all the way down to the ground, with an opening just large enough for a small child to climb into. I used to think the weeping willow could keep me safe from anything and imagined hiding in the heart of it.

The Petersons had five kids whose ages spanned about a ten-year period. From my perspective, there were two much older boys (Larry and Brad), one older girl (Anita), a girl a little older than me (Angie), and a girl a little younger than me (Denise).

When Angie was four or five she was hit by a car, and suffered significant brain injury. My mom says our family arrived at the scene of the accident shortly afterwards. I was about three. Angie never fully recovered, remaining physically awkward and severely mentally retarded, although quite sweet, for the rest of her life.

I liked Anita best and always wanted to hang out with her, probably because she was three years older and that made her cool by definition. I smoked my first pot with her and her friends. Anita got away from the family by getting married quite young. I thought the younger brother, Brad, was nice too, kind of quiet, very different from his older brother. Later, I heard his father didn't like him, because he didn't think Brad was biologically his.

Brad got pretty heavily into drugs as a young adult and had a heart attack at age 30. I don't remember too much about the youngest daughter, Denise, from my childhood. The mom, Marilyn, always looked tired, with deep purple bags under her eyes and sometimes bruises elsewhere. Even as a child I knew something was wrong.

The Petersons moved back east for a spell before returning to Washington State some years later. Not long after their return, the oldest brother Larry dived into a creek and broke his neck. I still remember visiting them when his hospital bed was set up in the middle of the dining room. He eventually recovered after a long convalescence. Even without probing too deeply beneath the surface, it was obvious that the Petersons had suffered greatly.

Still, Thanksgivings at their house were good times. Although their house was very small and always rather drab, it was quite cozy with all 11 of us in it when the smell of a traditional Thanksgiving feast filled it: turkey, gravy, mashed potatoes, and especially the cornbread. The women crowded into the tiny kitchen and cooked. The Petersons did not have a built-in dishwasher; at some point during the middle of the day Mrs Peterson would push a portable dishwasher into the tiny kitchen, hook it up to the faucet, and wash all the dishes, then move it back out of the way. Meanwhile, the men crowded into the small living room and watched football; a fire blazed and a large bowl of nuts sat on the hearth. I always made a beeline for the bowl of nuts. I loved the almonds and filberts best. I didn't have the patience to pick away the shell fragments from the pecans and walnuts, and I was not strong enough to crack open the Brazil nuts, but they fascinated me, and I used to make a game of watching to see who could crack a Brazil nut and pull the meat out whole.

As a child, the best part about those gatherings was that after dinner and a walk, we all played games together, and we kids got to stay up late. I enjoyed playing Totopoly, a horse racing and betting game with a two-sided board. On the first side, you purchased your horses and on the second side you raced them. It went on interminably. Sometimes we played Formula 1, a car racing game, or Tripoli, a betting card game that is sort of a combination of hearts, poker, and rummy. The adults drank heavily. At midnight, those still awake would have giant turkey sandwiches.

One Boxing Day we went to their house and learned that the older boys had received a BB gun for Christmas. This was exciting! All the kids gathered out in the backyard to watch them shoot it into the trees behind their house. Their backyard was unkempt grass that ended at a kind of dirt cliff that went steeply down and into a treed area. We were standing just over the edge on a dirt ledge, with the house behind us, and a small, forested area before us while the boys shot the BB gun. I must have been about seven. One of the boys turned and handed me the BB gun to hold. I found myself holding this gun with my finger wrapped around the trigger. Before I even thought about it, my finger instinctively pulled the trigger. Brad was actually peering into the end of the gun at that moment. I shot a BB into his eye. All of a sudden he was crying out and there was a flurry of activity with screaming and running. I still didn't really know what had happened. By a stroke of good fortune, the BB had hit the very corner of his eye only and did not do any lasting damage. I still wonder about that moment and why I pulled that trigger. It's the only time I have shot a gun.

These were my conscious childhood memories about our family and theirs. I was surprised when I began having flash-backs and visions that were considerably less benign and more terrifying. Where had these come from?

One time at a regional love and ecstasy meeting, we were in a group session when I told Jake that I had to leave the room. I was feeling prickly all over (I later came to associate this feeling with a sort of prescience that indicated a vision or flashback was coming). I asked Jake if he would come downstairs with me. We set up a more private sacred space and he began to work with me. Again, shortly after starting, I had another fragmented flashback. This scene took place in a bathroom. I could see bits and pieces that seemed to be Don Peterson masturbating. Then I was on his lap. I was very young, perhaps three or four, or so. Everything seemed to stop and shift, as if I were seeing the whole thing from the perspective of Don Peterson himself. I could feel his urgency, his keen desire to ejaculate, as he rubbed his penis between two young thighs. It was exciting, and even as I talked about the scene with Jake it made me aroused, which was very confusing. I could feel the primal energy in Mr Peterson's desire to come, while simultaneously feeling the horror of using a young child for one's own pleasure . . .

Still, the surfacing of these repressed memories triggered full-blown anxiety attacks. I wrote a poem about how such an anxiety attack feels:

Pounding in my chest
My tongue lies flat, heavy at the bottom of my mouth
My mouth tingles heavily
My teeth tingle
I can't feel my legs or anything beneath my mid-section

Tears pulse behind my eyes
Constricted breath

State of mind:
Narrow
Fearful
Racing
Wanting to control

Scared voice
Scared of being hurt
Protect self

This state of mind
Keeps me from being
Myself
I feel imprisoned in my body
It tells me I'm a fool

Stay tight, don't breathe, don't love, don't trust
The words whisper
Control
You must control, they insist

Arms tingling
Body trembling
Paralyzed
I feel paralyzed

From fear to emptiness, depression

Can't move, can't do
They whisper
Too heavy, too scared

You don't deserve to be happy – deserve?
Happiness is fleeting
There's no place to stand, nothing to lean against

Chapter 10

The Basement

O, full of scorpions is my mind . . .
~ Shakespeare

It was during one of the periods when we were home between love and ecstasy training cycles that I had the overwhelming feeling come over me to return to the neighborhood where I grew up. Some part of me knew this visit would further affect the course of my life. Up until this point, I could disbelieve my haunting visions, but what if they were real? What if they were verifiable? Was my childhood different from what I thought to be true?

I dropped my five-year-old daughter off at school and called my husband, Jake, from a payphone there. My body shook, heart pounding.

"Jake, I'm heading over to the Petersons' old house," I told him.

"Mariah, are you sure you want to go alone, now? Maybe I should come with you." His voice trailed off and I could sense his concern.

"I'm okay, Jake. I want to see this place. I have to. I'll call you later."

I hung up and stood for a moment gathering my courage, then drove to the lower middle-class neighborhood of Eastgate, Washington, where I had grown up. The houses were all smallish, mostly ramblers built in the 1950s with unkempt sickly lawns lining the street. I drove past my house, down the street two blocks, turned right and headed up the hill where I remembered Larry, the Petersons' oldest son, had practiced skateboarding, and where I had tried once and fell off. I drove past the house I thought was the Petersons' and around the other corner. Yep, we used to walk on this street after Thanksgiving dinner. I drove back to the house, parked, and then sat in my car staring at it. The paint was peeling and the driveway was potholed. Tall evergreen trees in the back shrouded the house in darkness. If the basement room I kept seeing in my visions was really there in that house, I couldn't tell from here. The shrubbery surrounding the house was overgrown, blocking any view into the backyard. I had last seen the Petersons more than 20 years ago, just before they moved away again. Whoever lived in the house now wouldn't know me. I paused. *I should probably leave*, I thought, but I'd come too far already and I needed to know.

I trembled as I imagined myself walking up to the front door and knocking, thinking what I might say: "Excuse me, um . . . I was just driving by and realized that this used to be a house that was an important part of my childhood. I was just wondering if I could look around, you know, for old times' sake . . . "

Oh my gads, that sounded pretty lame.

Then I watched, almost as if from a distance, as I actually got out of the car and walked up to the door and knocked.

Someone peered through the front window, then opened the door. To my surprise, it was Mrs Peterson, older, grayer, but still familiarly frumpy and easily recognizable. She had that same sad, haunted, and fatigued look I remembered, marked by sallow skin and dark purple circles under her eyes. Anita, her oldest daughter, now in her forties, stood next to her looking like a slightly plump soccer mom. What? I could barely speak for a moment or two. How could they be back there, 20 years later?

I looked up into the mother's eyes. "Hello. Do you remember me?"

"Yes. You're Mariah," she replied. "Come in. What brings you here?"

I entered the house, which was as depressing and dark on the inside as the outside, with tired, dog-eared, overstuffed, earthtone furniture, and worn, stained carpeting. I noted a faint stale smell.

"I . . . I don't really know where to start," I stammered. "I wasn't expecting to see you here. I thought you moved away."

"Yes," she replied. "We did, but we never sold it. We kept the house as a rental. We just moved back in, actually."

I digested these words, still feeling stunned. She continued, "So, fill us in. What about you? How are you?"

"Um . . . well, I am fine . . ." I said, dropping off at the end. I paused before pushing on.

Finally I said, "Look, I'm here because I have been having these flashbacks and dreams . . . and they're, well, they're somewhat disturbing, and they seem to be tied to this house."

Anita and her mother exchanged a look.

"Sit down," Mrs Peterson suggested. "Let me make you a cup of tea."

When she came back to the living room, I found I wasn't prepared to talk about the flashbacks, so instead I talked about my current life, that I was married and had two kids. That I'd lived in Los Angeles for a while before getting married, but now we were back in the area, and my brother was also married and had one child, and my folks were doing well, and so on.

I took a deep breath.

"The reason I am here is . . . well, I . . . I mean, my husband and I . . . um, well, we have been taking a kind of healing and meditation class," I began. "I've had these visions, I guess you could call them." I struggled with how to describe what had been going on with me.

Finally I blurted out, "I keep seeing some sort of dark, looming, evil-looking close-up of your husband, Don," I told Mrs Peterson, embarrassed by my confession. At the mention of his name, she and her daughter paled and jumped from the couch.

"Have you seen him?" Anita asked, agitation in her voice. "Is he here?"

Her mother moved to the windows and drew the front curtains.

"Uh . . . what? No. Not that I know of, anyway," I said. "Why?"

The two women looked at each other.

"Mom and Dad are divorced," Anita said. "We don't talk about him and we don't see him . . . ever. I have two children and I will not allow him to meet them."

"What? Really?"

"He is not a good person," she said and left it at that.

"I see." I sipped my tea, shaking now, my eyes silently filling with tears, then took a breath and began again.

"So, I've also had this vision or flash of a basement room, somehow tied with this house. It's confusing because your house is only one story, but in these visions, there is a dirt floor."

Mrs Peterson paused, then spoke slowly. "Actually, there is such a room in this house. It's the crawl space underneath, but it's quite big; you can stand up in it, if you are short. It's where we keep the washer and dryer. It has a dirt floor and there used to be an old mattress down there."

Silence filled the air.

"Would it be possible for me to look at it?" I asked hesitantly.

An inscrutable expression crossed Mrs Peterson's face, but then she shrugged and nodded.

We walked around the back of the house and I could see that the backyard sloped, creating extra space under the house; the main wall of the crawl space even had a small window. Around the side, there was a mini 4-foot-tall door of sorts. Mrs Peterson and Anita ducked through the doorway. I paused—suddenly terrified—then willed myself to continue. My body began shaking when I saw the washer and dryer standing to one side and a dirt floor. This was the room in my visions. Everything started to feel surreal.

Trembling uncontrollably, I felt weak and leaned on a wooden support post. I turned my attention left to the expanse of the room and remembered where the mattress had been—there between the posts. I couldn't look there. The edges of my vision blurred, and it felt like I was looking down a narrow tunnel. My eye was drawn to and focused instead on a bit of sunlight streaming through the small window, where it formed a small patch on the dirt floor. I hung on to that bit of light as if it were my sanity. What had happened to me here?

Mrs Peterson must have seen me grow pale and weak, because she said, "Let's go back inside," and the three of us fled from the underground room.

Sitting with these two women again, back in their dingy living room, I had so many questions, but I was afraid to voice them. What was that room used for? Why had there been a mattress down there? Why am I having visions about it? Why are you so scared at the mention of your ex-husband?

Instead, we tried to make a bit of small talk. It fell flat. I sat quietly sipping the last of my tea.

Finally, Mrs Peterson spoke up. "I know you have questions," she said, "but I am not the best person for you to talk to. You need to talk to Denise."

Anita nodded in agreement.

Denise? The youngest daughter? Why should I talk to her?

She continued, "Denise is working on a master's degree at the University of Washington. It would be better if you just talked to her." She handed Denise's number to me, but didn't offer any more information.

* * *

I don't remember leaving the house or driving home. My

thoughts dashed like rabbits this way and that, and a constant prickly creeping feeling rushed through my system. As soon as I got home, I called Jake to give him an update.

"Things are pretty weird," I said slowly.

"You sound funny," he replied. "Are you okay? Should I come home?"

"No, I'm okay. I know what I need to do."

Denise picked up on the first ring. She had not spoken to her mother or sister yet, so I had to explain who I was and why I was calling. I told her that prior to these visions, I had no conscious knowledge of anything untoward happening at all in my childhood.

She was quiet for a long moment, then spoke carefully.

"We need to talk."

I thought she meant in person, but instead she took a deep breath and began.

"It's hard to know where to start, but I'll try to fill you in. Let me say first, that your calling is a very strange coincidence. I'm currently getting my master's degree at the University of Washington in social work, and as part of my degree, I'm required to undergo some intense therapy sessions. At my last session yesterday, you came up very strongly for the first time. I was reliving part of my childhood and suddenly told my therapist that there was another child around. It was you. I told my therapist I felt scared for you." She paused.

My heart was beating fast. Did I hear her say that I just came up in her therapy session? How could she possibly have been thinking about me? We hadn't seen each other in over 20 years and weren't even close as kids.

"What are you saying?" I wished we were sitting face-to-face so I could see her.

"I'm saying that you were an important part of my last session."

"What does that mean?" I struggled to understand.

She went on, "You told me that you have been having strange visions or flashbacks that you don't understand. It sounds to me like you are having repressed memories surface."

I felt like she was talking about someone else. Repressed memories? Wait a minute. I had a happy childhood with loving parents. But Jake's words simultaneously echoed in my head: "How come you don't remember anything from when you were five or younger?" he'd asked. "Those are some of my favorite memories . . . playing with my dog, spending the days outside eating fruit off the trees." Could she be right? Could I have repressed certain memories?

Denise continued, "I have memories too, but most of mine were not repressed. I remember a lot because it went on for so long. Do you remember when we moved back east?" she asked.

I nodded, "Sort of. I learned at some point, after we moved to a different neighborhood, that you had moved away, out of state."

"Well, things were not good in our family. My dad terrified my mom and was always threatening to leave us. They would get in lots of fights and he would beat her. She would hide me in the closet, but it didn't always work. He beat and molested me too. When I was eight years old, my oldest brother, who was about nine years older than me, forced sex on me, too. I told my mom, but she didn't do anything."

Denise paused again and continued.

"One day, while we were living back east, my mom came home and said that our dad was leaving us for good. She was scared about how we would survive financially, but I immediately broke down on the floor sobbing, because it was the happiest day of my life."

Denise spoke calmly and deliberately as she relayed her story. She took a deep breath and kept on.

"Do you ever remember your vagina burning?" she asked.

"Um, I'm not sure," I responded, but even as I spoke I recalled a strange memory of persistent burning in my vagina as a child.

"Well, our mothers used to get together and talk and one day they both happened to find out that we were having similar symptoms of burning vaginas. They were trying to figure out what might have caused it. It didn't occur to them at the time that our burning vaginas were caused from matching sexual abuse."

Her words stung. I felt like a trapped animal. Questions were circling. Even with the strange flashbacks and the disturbing visit to the Peterson house, I hadn't truly accepted the idea that anything had *really* happened to me. Maybe I was just a sensitive kid and picked up on the experiences of others, or maybe I had witnessed something awful. Surely my parents would have known, my mom especially, if anything like that had happened to me.

How could I have been abused and not know until now?

Chapter 11

Weeds

You should rather be grateful for the weeds you have in your mind, because eventually they will enrich your practice.
~ Shunryu Suzuki

After visiting the basement and subsequently talking to Denise, I told everything to Jake, but it was difficult to know what to do. So, Jake and I went back to our lives and tried not to focus on the disturbing news I had heard from Denise. I was still a mess, however, and decided I should go to therapy. We had been once before for couple's therapy, but I wanted to go alone to investigate further what was happening to me. Mostly I was concerned about the trembling attacks that would overcome me and leave me incapacitated. I was still convinced that all of this really had to do with my shock at Jake's affair and that somehow I was conjuring up these flash images for sympathy or something.

The day I first drove to the therapist's office was a gray day, drizzling a little. The office was in a squat, two-story, 1970s-style brick building that leased space to all kinds of different small businesses. I sat in the car a bit before gathering up the courage to go inside.

I gave the receptionist my name and the name of the therapist and she took me back to a small room. I exchanged pleasantries with the therapist and she asked why I was there. As I started talking about what had happened with Jake and Shari, I got upset. Soon, I was crying uncontrollably and shaking all over.

The therapist seemed a little alarmed at my response and gave me a pillow to cry into. She said it might scare the people in the adjoining offices to hear me so upset. I thought that was strange, but cried into the pillow to muffle the sound. We had not talked about anything else yet, only the affair. After a bit, she said to me that she didn't think my reaction was only about an affair. She said she thought I had PTSD. I didn't know what that was, so she elaborated: post-traumatic stress disorder. Was there anything that had happened in my childhood that might have caused me stress?

I sat there in shock, unsure how to proceed. Even with everything that I had been through and with Denise telling me all that she had told me too, I still somehow didn't believe anything had happened. So when she asked me if my childhood had had any trauma, it felt almost like lying to say yes. It wasn't like I perfectly remembered anything traumatic . . . I said I didn't know for sure, but that I had been having these strange flashbacks and had learned some disturbing information about family friends. She suggested that we take one of the images and work with it. She said we would start slow and she would help me not to get too overwrought.

"First," she said, "just think about one of the partial images from these flashbacks. Don't worry about if it makes sense. Just describe what you see. I am right here."

I closed my eyes and began haltingly.

"I was sleeping on the floor in one of the bedrooms . . . I woke up, I guess . . . and I . . . I walked across the little hallway . . . into the bathroom . . . Everyone else was asleep . . . I was so little . . . Don Peterson was in there and . . . and . . . then I was sitting on his lap . . . and . . . Mommy! —"

The therapist abruptly brought me out of the scene.

"Did you hear what you were saying?" she asked. "You were calling out for your mommy. You sounded like a very young child. This is not an anxiety attack caused solely by what happened with your husband and your friend. This is deeper than that."

As she calmed me down, she said again that what I was experiencing was classic PTSD, and that my reactions to the affair were much too strong for that to be the only cause. For the first time, I began to allow the possibility that I had experienced childhood trauma. It seemed completely improbable to me that she would come up with the idea, without having known anything about the visions and flashbacks and backstory. The fact that she came up with it independently, combined with the empirical evidence from visiting the house and talking to Denise, combined with the strange flashback visions, finally allowed the notion to set in.

I continued to work with the therapist for a bit. We talked about other memories from my childhood that I could recall. I began telling her one odd story, almost as if from rote. It had been a part of my memory banks, but strangely I had never examined it in detail. In the story, I had been playing horsey on a wooden broomstick. Somehow I slipped and hurt myself. I called out for my mother and she took me to the doctor. The doctor said my hymen was broken. The therapist questioned me quite a bit about the incident: Was I wearing underwear? Did the stick penetrate me? Was there blood? I could not recall any of these things and neither could my mother, when I asked her later. The story didn't make sense.

The therapist wanted to try out a new technique called EMDR (eye movement desensitization and reprocessing), which involves rapid eye movement, thought to lessen the effect of PTSD. I eventually did an EMDR session with her, but then had to stop therapy, because our insurance changed and the sessions were no longer covered.

I never did get around to telling her some other things that I later learned were common for people who had repressed memories of sexual abuse. I learned these from a book called

Repressed Memories: A Journey to Recovery from Sexual Abuse, by Renee Frederickson. It contained a symptom checklist. The first two lines of the checklist read: "1) I began masturbating at a very early age," and "2) As a child I used to insert objects into my bottom, and do not know where I learned to do this." That stopped me cold, because both of these were true for me, although I didn't know they were unusual. I did start masturbating at a young age and my favorite form of masturbation involved using broken pencils with the sharp end inserted into my vagina or rectum, or preferably both . . . I didn't learn to masturbate lying on my back using my fingers until attending the love and ecstasy training. I had always lain on my stomach with objects inserted inside me, and a heavy blanket applying pressure.

Although my talk therapy sessions had ended, Jake and I continued to attend Margot Anand's program and continued to practice the myofascial pelvic release practices at home. These proved to be extraordinarily powerful techniques. There was no doubt that I was releasing toxic memories. Eventually, an odd symptom directly related to various release sessions began to appear. This first happened the day after a particularly strong session—a session that triggered a PTSD/anxiety response. When I awoke the morning after, I found a ring of tiny blisters completely encircling each of my wrists, as if the wrists had been tied or somehow restrained. This was hugely disturbing, as I didn't have any conscious memory of being restrained, but still my body seemed to. The blistering around the wrists only happened once, but other tiny blisters, generally on my hands and fingers, sometimes appeared following release sessions. We came to count on that as an indication that we had successfully released something, and while it was scary to go through, it was also encouraging; healing was happening. My body seemed to remember more than I ever would, perhaps because whatever had happened, had happened when I was very young—under five.

I worried that the stress would be too much for our shaky relationship. We had read that two of the most difficult things a couple can go through were infidelity and PTSD from abuse, and here we were dealing with both.

One day I was resting on our bed when Jake walked in.

"I was looking through the books at Barnes and Noble today and came across this one," he said, handing me a book. "I thought it was perfect for us."

The book was *I Will Never Leave You*, by Hugh and Gayle Prather. I was deeply touched. Hugh and Gayle were renowned couples counselors and best-selling authors who presented a detailed program for saving any relationship and helping it become permanent, satisfying, and spiritually centered. They argued that breaking up was seldom the best solution for a troubled marriage. I remember little of the book's contents, but I will never forget the moment when Jake handed me that book, nor the message his doing so gave me: these were hard times, but we would work hard and get through them, together.

True to that promise, Jake was unbearably sweet and endlessly patient with me during this time, which is why I never felt like I needed more therapy, despite the intensity. He held me often and comforted me. He told me "Everything will be okay," which were words I never tired of hearing and which I believed when he said them. He held my gaze with deep, soul-penetrating eyes when things got rough for me. I felt cradled by his presence, much as I had during that first experience with the snake vision. He made me feel like I was the most important thing going on in his life and like this difficult journey through the recovery of these memories was something we were doing together. His presence and support during this process overshadowed any hurt feelings I had from the affair, and I relaxed into trusting him again.

Jake's most important gift to me, however, was that he never saw or treated me as a victim. He was influenced from the start by the first spiritual book we read—the one recommended by the makeup lady at the television program: *Zen Mind, Beginner's Mind*, by Shunryu Suzuki. Suzuki said, "For Zen students a weed . . . is a treasure." Jake held that light up for me over and over again. He would say, when things got tough, "These memories are just grist and weeds for the enlightenment wheel. And the deeper and more prevalent the weeds, the more beautiful and fertile the soil when we expose them."

For a time, we worked to see if we could extract more specific memories, but never got much beyond fragmented visuals. We were guided by my visceral responses, however, and would work together to allow feelings to come up, to be experienced, and to pass on. The pelvic release sessions that we learned during love and ecstasy training were supremely powerful and effective in releasing trapped memories and creating an opening to heal.

There was something freeing about simply feeling afraid or sad without judging it. It was the start of a journey where, in the long run, I would come to appreciate that traveling to the basement of my mind and cleaning the darkest closets, exposing and accepting my most vulnerable self, ultimately empowered and freed me. My greatest fear had been that my feelings were stronger than I was, but again and again, I have dived into my deep, ugly feelings, felt humiliation and shame, cried buckets, been afraid, and then inexplicably moved on, free to feel the next feeling, which could just as easily be joy or love.

I learned a lot during this era and came to trust that feelings will pass. One day, as I was crying in front of my five-year-old daughter, she sweetly looked at me and said, with a child's instinctive wisdom what I was just learning to be true: "Don't worry, Mommy, if you feel sad right now, because the next feeling you feel will be something else, like glad!"

All during this time, Jake was there for me, and I recognized his commitment. I also knew he had his own demons to battle, which came up a bit during our training, but which he did not fully face until much later. He had been severely bullied as a teenager and had himself been molested by an older cousin. Plus, his family had a history of serious depression. His grandfather on his father's side had committed suicide, as had three of his uncles and one cousin. Jake had tried medication but didn't like its dulling effect on his body and mind; more importantly, he believed medication would hinder enlightenment and that with awareness practice one could also escape from depression.

Jake's inner struggle was intermittent and ultimately would take much longer coming to a head. Unlike me, who thrived on his support during times of personal crisis, when he was troubled, he would push me away and retreat into a cave to battle his demons on his own. But that was to come later . . .

Chapter 12

Multi-Orgasmic Response – MORE

When the marriage between energy and consciousness happens at the level of the heart, there is a heart orgasm; when the marriage happens at the level of the third eye, the energy expands beyond the boundaries of the body and you experience spaciousness, a lightness . . . When the orgasmic energy of pleasure is channeled all the way to the sahasrara chakra, the receiver becomes one with all that is; it is access to bliss.

~ Margot Anand

Meanwhile, our love and ecstasy training continued, and, after three months, we moved into the second session, which included a section called, much to our delight, "MORE," for multi-orgasmic response.

The goal of MORE is to expand one's orgasmic potential. It is the heart of what people tend to think of when Tantra is mentioned: extended lovemaking sessions. In the MORE sessions, we learned about the importance of communication. People are inclined to believe that since sex is so natural, everything should always be spontaneous, and that verbal communication is not necessary. We learned that it is important to spend some significant time and effort learning to communicate details with your partner, to learn how to bring your partner pleasure.

We focused first on one person's pleasure, the receiver, and then switched roles. As the giver moved from one spot to another, they might ask, "How does this feel? How about this?

What about when I move faster? Or slower?" The giver would ask permission, such as, "Is it okay if I push harder?" or "I am going to try this move; let me know how it feels." This kind of detailed sexual communication feels awkward at first, but is invaluable later. It taught us to tune in to the subtleties of both giving and receiving pleasure. Generally, when the questions are being asked you are gazing at one another, and there is a wonderful feeling of connection as you deliberately explore together the receiver's body.

Also, by this point in the training, Margot had done a number of exercises to get us to open up the "inner flute," which might be described as an energy channel that runs between chakras or energy centers at various points in the body. The inner flute is well known in many other traditions and has many names: the Central Channel, Sushumna, the inner reed, the hollow bamboo, the path of Kundalini, to name a few. Prior to taking Margot's class, however, I did not know about any of these, nor did I know anything about chakras. It all sounded esoteric, strange, and unlikely. Nevertheless I came to appreciate that different energy centers do exist and that there is an energy channel running between them that I could experience for myself, particularly during lovemaking.

Once we started to practice MORE sessions, we came to appreciate the potential love and ecstasy exercises had, not only to expose and heal traumatic memories, but also to replace them with extraordinary blissful ones. We began to relearn everything we thought we knew about sex.

There is a difference, for instance, between what I came to think of as a peak orgasm and a valley orgasm. A peak orgasm is what we experience in a typical Western sexual encounter. It is focused on the genitals and is dependent on the active build-up of excitement. It is a quick rush reached through extreme tension to orgasm. It is good. It is therapeutic. It is relieving of sexual tension. It is also goal oriented. During peak-orgasm sex, you focus on getting to climax, and as wonderful as it is, you can miss a whole plethora of subtler joys, of intimacy, of connection and union . . . of extended bliss.

A valley orgasm is different. It happens when you relax while in a state of high arousal. You maintain the high arousal without peaking, by using certain breathing techniques, doing intentional pelvic contractions, and bringing awareness to the act. You work with your partner to notice what the other is experiencing and back off or engage further to prolong the energy that is building. The experience includes the genitals, and genital stimulation is key to getting started, but ultimately the experience includes the whole body as energy moves in waves up your body and reaches your heart region. Although I would never normally be aware of any feeling of tension or holding in the chest region, when the energy passes through, it feels as if the heart completely relaxes and melts. It is difficult to describe but there is an exquisite feeling of complete surrender combined with intense compassion and love. Often I cry out of gratitude for life at this stage. Often I feel like I travel to some other realm—my mind lets go and I feel like my consciousness is floating in a warm deep space—aware of but untethered to the physical body. The intimacy or connection with Jake, with whom I am still soul gazing, is astounding. The feeling lasts much longer and is ultimately much more deeply satisfying than what *Men's Health* magazine penned "the normal six-second genital sneeze." When a couple simultaneously reaches this type of extended, whole-body orgasm, it is called "Riding the Wave of Bliss," and once you experience it, you will not forget it, nor will you be satisfied with ordinary, goal-oriented sex—though, of course, you can still enjoy "quickies" too.

Jake and I were more than a little titillated to practice all that we were learning from pelvic release to the Wave of Bliss, to playful lover's games at home. One of our favorite games was called the Yin Yang (or Master/Servant) game. In it, we each took turns for an agreed-upon period of time—say one or two hours—practicing perfect surrender as the Yin (Servant) party to the other's Yang (Master), who called the shots. The Yang party could ask for *anything* during the designated period of time and the Yin party sweetly, lovingly, without argument complied. If by chance the Yang party asked something that the Yin party truly felt was outside their ability or comfort zone to deliver, the appropriate response would be, "Please, master, I am so sorry to disappoint you. I cannot comply with your wishes. Is there anything else I can do for you?" Thirteenth-century Persian poet and Sufi mystic, Rumi, underscores the power of this very game. In one poem he writes in part about a couple who appeared happier than others. In it he says "Their secret was: That once every day for an hour they would treat each as if they were gods, and would do anything, anything their beloved asked" (Rumi, "Their Secret Was," translated by Daniel Ladinsky).

We had always been good students and now we had "sex homework," which added a playful element to our normal suburban routine, despite the difficult challenges we were facing. Together, we carved time out to practice whenever we could. Life in the bedroom became anything but boring. A door to more had been opened.

We had been through a lot together, having faced infidelity, intense group therapy, and the sudden unexpected occurrence of crushing repressed memories. Even as we appreciated the intro-duction to meditation and the extraordinary sexual practices we had learned, however, we knew our healing wasn't complete. A door to more may have been opened, but it was up to us now to keep practicing, and we vowed to do so. We also knew instinc-tively that we needed a reprieve. We sought to escape for a spell, somewhere far from home, somewhere we could heal, somewhere we could integrate and process, somewhere off the beaten track.

Part II

The Respite

Chapter 13

Yelapa

Allow time to integrate. You've learned a lot. Take time. Give yourself space.
~ Margot Anand

Morning greeted us quietly with stars fading to planets, finally giving way to a rosy sunrise over the river while we did our yoga and meditated from the tiny casita that overlooked the bay. I wrote in my journal,

> Dawn's light illuminated new channels in the river carved by the night's surf. Flocks of white birds, perhaps Snowy Egret, circled over the river like the mad thoughts that chased around in my brain. Sometimes I feel my mind quiet amidst the paradox that makes up Yelapa.
> (Journal entry, January 1997)

Yelapa was classic paradise: white sandy beaches, coconut trees, lush foliage, romantic, thatch-roofed *palapas*, and clear ocean water. It's just that it was hell, too: scorpions hiding in shoes and closets, polluted drinking water, the smell of burning plastic, fear of disease, and horse caca everywhere.

Our mid-life crisis, or perhaps I should call it mid-life awakening, brought our family here. A friend we made during the training offered us the chance to live in her palapa for three months in this remote fishing village south of Puerto Vallarta. It sounded perfect. Yelapa, we decided—a place where heaven and hell co-existed over the rubble of prior earthquakes—was our place to integrate. Winter 1997—when heaven and hell co-existed in the rubble of our hearts—was our time to integrate. Our stint in Yelapa was a grand and crazy adventure from the start, rather like Monty Python's "And now for something completely different . . . "

We took an extended sabbatical from work, rented our house to friends, and—imagining we might just stay forever, living cheap on the beach, never working again—left on one-way tickets for Mexico at the tail end of one of the most severe snowstorms ever to hit the Pacific Northwest. We planned this to be a reprieve of the grandest sort—off the beaten track with completely different concerns confronting us. We wanted this to be an opportunity for our whole family to play together. Of course, we would come to learn that wherever you go, there you are, but for a time we focused only on the very different problems of moving to a remote village in Mexico with two young children. We allowed ourselves the opportunity to get swept away in the newness of everything. We saw it as a chance to start fresh, using as a foundation our joint love of adventure, first shared so long ago when we made our driftwood and kelp raft. This was an opportunity for us to create a new story together far from the cry of infidelity and abuse.

We arrived in Puerto Vallarta with the following simple instructions from our friend: "Go down to the big beach and ask for a *panga* going to Yelapa. When you arrive in Yelapa, just ask where Josie's house is. Everybody will know."

Soon, we found ourselves standing on a beach in Puerto Vallarta armed with rough traveler's Spanish, seven enormous suitcases, two kids, and two kittens, gazing out to sea. "*Dondé está la panga a Yelapa?*" we asked. "*Está alla,*" someone responded, pointing out to sea.

A *panga*, it turned out, was a smallish—about 20 feet long—open-aired, outboard-powered boat with a high bow, a fiberglass-coated wooden hull, and a narrow waterline beam. It pretty much looked like an extra long rowboat with a motor and seats. The pangas couldn't come all the way to shore, and there was no dock to walk out on. We stood there, trying to figure out our next move, and were encouraged when a couple of strong young men grabbed our belongings, carried them out and piled them into one of the pangas. I was beginning to wonder how we were going to get the stuff out there.

There were lots of other people standing around on the beach with their luggage, too. The men grabbed all their stuff and piled it into the panga, too. I watched the gunwale sink lower and lower. There were other pangas about, so I assumed one would carry the baggage and another would carry us. Wrong. After 20 people's significant luggage had been loaded, the men indicated that the people should load too. The boat was absolutely packed from bow to stern and every spare bit of the floor taken. We perched precariously on one of the wooden benches, the two kids between us, the cats in a carry case at our feet.

Without further ado, we got underway. It began to dawn on me as I looked around that this was the most unsafe thing I had ever done. "Jake," I whispered urgently, "there are no life jackets! Look how close the water is to flowing over the edge. Jake, we have to dig out our BCs and put them on the kids."

Jake located our luggage somehow and dug for the scuba gear we'd brought with us. A buoyancy jacket or BC is not a life jacket exactly, but at least it inflates and offers some support. We put them on the kids, who looked dwarfed in them, and huddled back on our seats. There was a wild-eyed young man sitting next to me who looked like he spoke English.

"Hey," I said nervously. "How are you doing? Do you live in Yelapa?"

He said "Yeah, sometimes. I am just returning. I've been away for a while."

"Oh, really? So what's it like?"

"Oh, it's really great. Beautiful, you know. A bunch of my friends live there and we hang out at the beach a lot."

"Nice," I responded.

Our friend Josie had told us there were several different cultures, both gringo and native, in Yelapa. There were the artist/hippy types who tended to live super cheap and hang out on the beach, generally high or drunk; there were the expatriated professionals, who spent a good portion of each year in Yelapa on sabbatical from their regular jobs; and there was the native population, made up mostly of fisherman and their families with a few shopkeepers and restaurant owners. Much as hanging out with hippies appealed to a younger side of me, we hoped to hook up with the professional expatriates, and I hoped some of them had kids.

I gathered that the young man next to me was more of the artist/hippy type, but I decided to ask the question that was really on my mind. "Sooo," I started, half chuckling to indicate I was kind of joking, "how often do these pangas sink?"

"Oh. I don't know," he responded. "Probably not more than one or two each year."

What? my brain screamed silently. *What do you mean, one or two a year?* I had been expecting something more along the lines of "Oh, don't worry. These things are really safe. These guys know what they're doing!"

I gulped. "So, they do turn over sometimes, huh?"

"Yeah. But you know, usually they aren't too far from shore."

I looked around at my two little kids and our cats and thought frantically, *How far out would I have to be? That would be disastrous . . . How well can the kids swim?*

I sat there for a bit, then tried to engage in further conversation to lessen my nerves.

"So, why did you leave? Were you called away to do something somewhere else for a while? It must have been hard to leave paradise, huh?"

"Oh no," he said. "It wasn't like that. There was an outbreak of typhoid fever. I wanted to get out of there."

"Typhoid fever?" I stammered.

"Yes. It was a rough year for Yelapa, because, of course, that eight-year-old girl also died from the scorpion bite earlier."

"Scorpion bite?" My mind was reeling. My God, what had we gotten ourselves into? I hugged my seven-year-old daughter tighter to me and wondered how much longer the boat trip was going to last and whether we could just turn around once we got there.

"But you're going back," I finally offered, looking for the silver lining.

"Yep. Yelapa is somethin' special. She's beautiful. Paradise really. Once you've tasted her, she's hard to forget. Just make sure you boil your water and don't stick your hands into any dark corners! You'll be fine."

Funny thing is, I don't think he even registered that he was freaking me out. For him, it was all par for the course.

Eventually, we landed near a little beach and I breathed a big sigh of relief. The guys helped us unload our seven massive bags that held everything we needed to live for the next three months: clothes, toiletries, reading books, schoolbooks, toys, scuba-diving gear, first-aid kits, a few specialty food items. We'd brought our four-month-old kittens with us as a kind of bribe for the kids. We figured if they were focused on taking care of their little kittens they wouldn't focus so much on themselves. And it worked, too! Our little four-year-old Cassie was cooing at the cats and telling them not to worry, everything would be okay. The hard part was over.

So there we were, two adults, two little kids, two kittens, and all our luggage on a new beach. We looked up at our totally unfamiliar surroundings in awe. The land rose steeply from the beach in most directions. Palm trees dotted the sand. There was no town visible, only the tips of thatched roofs peaking out from dense jungle foliage. Our awe gave way after a few minutes to practicality; it was time to make our way to our *casita*, or house. We had asked our friend for the address, but she kind of laughed. "Oh, there are no addresses in Yelapa," she relied. "But," she went on, "don't worry. It's on the hill to the right of the little beach. Just ask the first person you see 'Where is Josie's house?' They will know and take you there."

While the kids worried over the cats, Jake headed up the beach a bit to get directions from a man standing there. There was some exchange and then Jake headed back. He shook his head. The guy didn't know. Jake ran after about ten different folks. None of them had heard of "Josie's house." I stood there thinking how ridiculous the scene was—all the bags tossed about on the beach and us having no clue where we were or where we were going. About that time, a couple of strapping young guys came over to us and offered to carry our luggage. We still didn't know where we were going, but we also didn't want to be stranded on the beach carrying our kids and the luggage as it got dark.

Jake motioned to the guys to carry the luggage and said, "I'll run up the trail and see if I can figure out which house it is. She said it was somewhere on this hill. I can ask people as we go. Someone must know Josie. You come along with the kids and cats. You can just go slow." So we took off: me carrying one bag, the kids each taking one strap of the kittens' carrycase and the three young Mexican lads managing the rest of the giant suitcases. They would hoist one up onto a shoulder, balancing it between their shoulder and neck and carry another in their free hand. We learned later that they were so strong and capable because they made their living hand-carrying propane tanks on their shoulders to all the individual casitas that dotted the hills.

The path was dirt and rubble strewn and dotted with horse manure and other animal droppings. It twisted and winded and most definitely went *up*. Galvanized water pipes were draped haphazardly all over the hillside, frequently and dangerously crossing the trail. Jake ran up ahead and tried to talk to someone at every casita he came to. He zigzagged up and back and up and back, leaving us a breadcrumb trail of houses that were *not* Josie's house. Eventually, a considerable time and many houses and inquiries later, he came running back and said he'd found it. He explained, "There was an empty casita up the road. I went all the way into it and found a note there that Josie left for us. Come on! It's this way!"

Our place comprised two casitas, one slightly larger than the other and including a kitchen and dining area. These casitas were made palapa-style, which essentially meant they had concrete floors, half walls, and thatch roofs. No doors, no windows. No floor-to-ceiling walls. Everything was open air. Beds enshrouded in mosquito netting hung suspended from the rafters. The master bedroom was a loft overlooking the kitchen/living area, reached by a handmade ladder of tree limbs, polished shiny from use. The rest of the furnishings were simple: the basic kitchen essentials, the most important of which was a giant pot for boiling water, a table and four chairs, and a cement bench topped with a piece of foam and attached to one of the half walls that served as our "couch." Wooden stumps with pieces of branches sticking out served to hold up the roof and provided hooks for our jackets. There were a couple of hammocks strung between openings in the half walls. The place looked like something straight out of *Robinson Crusoe*. It was enchanting, for sure, but it offered almost no protection from what was going to be the coldest winter Yelapa had seen for over 20 years. We hadn't packed for cool weather. I had one sweater with me that I had to wear almost every day. The Mexicans, we learned, didn't inhabit the romantic-looking palapas we gringos were attracted to. They all lived in unattractive cement houses that offered protection from the elements and from the abundant critters that lived in Yelapa.

Still, we were happy. At last we had found our home-away-from-home. But that first night was intense; with no enclosed walls to insulate us from the experience, we felt exposed and vulnerable. Yelapa is a confluence of sounds and habitats. It is a town on the edge of the ocean, accessible only by boat, thrust up against the mountainous jungle. A symphony of braying donkeys, mooing cows, barking dogs, crowing roosters, cats in heat, and rummaging raccoons constantly assailed our ears. The roar of the ocean and the singing of thousands of cicadas accompanied that bunch. The birds of Yelapa were particularly memorable. All sorts flocked on the breezes that swirled through the river-lined canyon on the way out to sea: seagulls, parakeets, frigate birds, pelicans, woodpeckers, blue birds, red birds, humming birds, snowy egrets.

At the time we were there, there were no cars, no personal phones, and no electricity in Yelapa, although we did have the luxury of propane stoves and flush toilets. The town had only one phone and one fax machine. There were three tiny grocery stores, one little bakery, a kindergarten, and a handful of restaurants. One nurse and one doctor provided the only medical care in town, but unfortunately, the doctor was also the town drunk.

Yelapa is situated around a large, protected bay. At the north end, and at the far side of the bay from where we stayed, was the "tourist beach." A ferryboat brought tourists to this beach on day trips from Puerto Vallarta every day. The tourist beach was a swath of sandy beachfront that included a small hotel and low-key beach restaurants. It was a funky kind of hippy/artist beach scene with music always playing. At the edge of the tourist beach closest to town, a large river met the sea, bisecting the pathway separating the tourist beach from the rest of Yelapa. The silty banks of the river provided much entertainment as the flow changed daily. Sometimes the river crossing was narrow and only ankle deep; others times it was a block wide and shoulder deep.

On our end of the bay, there was another little beach where the water-taxi pangas and fishermen launched their boats. This was the beach we had first landed upon. Further on down to the south and along the coastline away from town, the hillside was dotted with a multitude of casitas. Our casita was about a 10-minute walk to town and the river crossing another 10 or 15 minutes further along. The trail leading to the river was haphazard at best and climbed along the cliff side next to the jungle, through ruins and over rubble. Then we had to cross the river to reach the tourist beach—always an exciting prospect with two young children. From the farthest residence south to the tip of the tourist beach was about an hour walk.

We spent much of every day walking, and we relished the physical exercise. On any given day we'd spend half of it traveling to and from our casita: going to the beach to play with the kids; to the store or a restaurant multiple times for food; to visit with various people; to hike up the mountain or to the waterfall. We got in great shape. Life was simple, but not necessarily easy.

Much as we relished these beautiful new memories and funny stories we were creating, there were still intense feelings pulsing under the surface from the last year and a half of life. Everything I thought I knew about myself had been tossed into the wind. My self-esteem rested on shaky grounds. I used to walk through the world thinking of myself as a cheerful, confident, capable, and loving person, but I no longer knew if those descriptions applied. How would I define myself now? Was I a victim? Was I light-hearted and easy-going, or difficult and unpredictable? Did I have unconscious programs running? Was I even lovable?

With no job or shopping or errand-running to distract us, we found ourselves with plenty of time in Yelapa. One of the hardest parts of life there was overcoming boredom. We spent time every day homeschooling and I had a creative outlet in painting and tie dyeing, but Jake had nothing. Back home, his usual relaxing outlet was to work in the yard, but this yard did not belong to us and did not require any care. Jake had a tendency to sink into depression, and with little else to distract him, our beautiful surroundings alone did not perfectly alleviate that. As I was mulling over who I was, Jake, too, was struggling.

One day early in our stay, Jake refused to get out of bed. He lay in the loft, projecting a field of darkness and despair. Suddenly, there was a loud raucous noise on the thatched roof above his head: a "wake," that is, a group of big black vultures like those from the kids' movie *Jungle Book* had landed just above his head. They remained there for hours. It certainly felt like they were waiting for him to die, so as to get on with devouring his carcass. In the end though, their presence seemed so amusing and ridiculous to Jake that it put him in a different frame of mind. I asked what happened to bring him out of his funk. He said that while he was lying there he suddenly remembered that during love and ecstasy training meditation and yoga had helped his depression.

"Let's wake up early every day as the sun rises and do yoga and meditation in the casita before the kids get up," he suggested.

I loved this idea and it came to be one of my most cherished memories from our stay in Yelapa. I read later that in earth-based spiritual traditions, the vulture confirms a new relationship between the volatile and fixed aspects of life, between psychic energies and cosmic forces. The appearance of a vulture can be considered a promise that suffering is temporary and necessary for a higher purpose, even if not understood at the time.

The decision to wake each morning with the sunrise and to practice meditating and yoga gave our stay in Yelapa a new focus. It changed the dynamic of the day and gave us a few moments to ourselves before we got busy taking care of the kids. It also made us realize that we needed some grown-up time, too. We began reaching out to others who were staying there, hopeful to meet some families with kids. We did meet a wonderful couple, who had a son, Bodhi, just a year older than Jacki, our oldest daughter, and they became fast friends. We were able to swap play dates. We decided to enroll Cassie in the local kindergarten, so that she might have an opportunity to meet other kids her age and to learn Spanish.

We began to meet more adults, too, who all had interesting stories and backgrounds. One couple, who practiced Ayurvedic medicine, offered all kinds of Ayurvedic treatments right there in Yelapa. Ayurveda is a Hindu system of medicine, which uses diet, herbal treatment, and yogic breathing. Jake signed up for Shirodhara, a special treatment where warm oil is dripped on the forehead to soothe and invigorate the senses and the mind. Another new acquaintance had studied Sufi dancing and offered a Sufi-dancing circle one night. One woman had come to Yelapa with her four kids aged 4 to 16 after her husband died. She, like us, had needed time and space to integrate. She decided while there to go back to school to study forensics. We got together with her and her kids sometimes to play games.

We wanted to share some of what we had learned too, and came up with the idea of offering a Tantra workshop for some of the couples we had met. We put together a program that focused on the importance of communication. In a sweet little casita perched on a cliff overlooking the ocean, we did an exercise where one partner massaged only the face of the other. With each subtle and gentle movement the one receiving would tune in and describe how it felt.

We began to appreciate and get in tune, too, with the sleepy, slow rhythm of living in Yelapa. It was such a contrast to suburban or urban life in America. In many ways, Yelapa felt safe and protected. We could encourage our four- and seven-year-old girls to walk on their own to the store, for instance. There were no cars, no weirdo predators potentially lurking. We would give them a few pesos and they would go to the local candy shop for treats, learning how to count in the process. The shopkeepers loved our little blonde-haired, blue-eyed angels. And we liked shopping in their stores, all the size of our kitchen, and with little more than one of everything. If one store was out, we wandered on down to the next one. There were no endless decisions to make as to which brand of beans to buy. Most of what we ate was fresh: papayas, mangos, coconuts, avocados off the tree, cilantro, basil, jalapenos, tomatoes out of gardens. Fresh-baked muffins and hibiscus tea, made from local blossoms. Handmade corn tortillas daily. Fish caught locally that day. The food was simple but sublime. "I could live here," I wrote to my family and friends after three weeks. "I like this lifestyle."

But everything was not bliss, for, like us, Yelapa had scorpions in her closets, and we had to learn how to deal with those, too.

Chapter 14

Dancing with Scorpions

When scorpions appear in our life, it symbolizes dynamic transformation through secret passions and desires . . . Unless we control our passions and desires and direct their energies appropriately, the transformations will occur in the midst of chaos.

~ Ted Andrews

Scorpions became the theme that wove through our entire stay. We didn't have a computer or Internet, but we learned from the locals that there were three types of scorpions in the Yelapa region: black, yellow, and black-and-yellow. The black ones were the mildest and although their sting was very painful, it was not deadly; the black-and-yellow ones were more poisonous; the yellow ones were really nasty. We learned later they were called "bark scorpions" and are among the deadliest variety of scorpions in the world and the most venomous in North America. Although the United States has registered only four scorpion-related deaths over 11 years, Mexico has experienced about 1000 reported deaths from the bark scorpion every year. The sting of the bark scorpion causes loss of muscle control and difficulty in breathing, and can be deadly to children or old people, who tend to have more severe reactions.

Many of our homeschooling lessons had a scorpion theme, as we got up to speed on these creatures. Research: "Let's study scorpions and learn about their habitat. We can read books and talk to the locals," I'd say. Writing: "Make a report that tells everything you know about scorpions." Presentation: "Create a poster outlining the main ways to avoid a scorpion." Science: "If we see a scorpion, we can kill it and preserve it in alcohol to study it a little closer."

Having heard the story about the eight-year-old girl who had died from a scorpion bite, we became diligent about keeping a look out for these critters. No clothes could be left on the ground. All shoes had to be shaken out before stepping into them. No reaching into cupboards. No sitting on the couch without lifting the cushion first. This was a major step beyond "Don't touch a hot stove." There was no room for mistakes. At first, we imagined that we might not see any scorpions, that they were extremely rare, but we actually saw half a dozen or so during our stay. We learned, however, that despite the prevalence of scorpions, there was a certain inherent natural balance to the environment, and that Yelapa had a couple of secret weapons for dealing with them. If we hadn't appreciated the danger, however, we might never have appreciated the beauty of the solutions.

One of these natural solutions to the scorpion problem came in the form of armies of ants that roamed the area. Yelapa was essentially a rubble-strewn anthill. There were all kinds of ants, whose names I never learned, but I can tell you that whether the individual ants were large or small, the colony operated the same way, which was unlike anything I had ever seen before. I was used to ants that hovered on or near their anthill and sent out scouts to forage for food that might eventually cause a line of ants to follow the trail to the source of the food—generally human food. But these ants foraged differently. They traveled in enormous armies that might stretch 30 to 100 feet wide—a mass of moving blackness. They would march up the hill across the footpath and right on through your house. The first time we saw this we were horrified.

The girls were each on a hammock when they looked down and screamed for us. When we came into the kitchen you couldn't even see the floor for the mass of moving blackness. We grabbed the girls and dashed out of the casita. We ran into a local and started to describe in panicky voices what we had seen. He started laughing and described in Spanish and broken English that this was a good thing: "*Se trata de un día para jugar en la playa!*" he said. "It is a day to go to the beach!"

We learned that Yelapans loved the ant armies and that any day an ant army arrived was immediately declared a vacation. Everyone left their home or work and went off to play elsewhere while the ants did the dirty work. These carnivorous ants traveled over every surface of the house, every nook, every cranny, and devoured other ants, cockroaches, beetles, moths, spiders . . . and scorpions, not to mention crumbs and spills. After an ant army had been through your house, it was immaculate. Who would have thought! We learned quickly, and when an ant army appeared to be headed for our casita, we simply went to the beach.

But our favorite Yelapan secret weapon was another creature altogether, called a "scorpion eater." They are gigantic alien-looking spiders, 7 to 10 inches in diameter, with strange, long legs that keep their body raised many inches above the ground, and what appear to be pincers at the front. They are nocturnal, like scorpions, and, as you might suspect from the name, are beloved by humans because they eat scorpions. In Yelapa, it is considered a huge blessing to have a resident scorpion eater in your house, as we did. So I got used to passing by the shelves where the scorpion eater, who was as big as a dinner plate, lived. She became almost like a pet. Thank you, scorpion eater. Good scorpion eater. We love you, scorpion eater. Life is strange that way.

The scorpions in the closets and hidden corners of Yelapa became symbolic to me of the scorpions hiding in my own mind. I came to appreciate that a certain diligence and care was needed in cleaning out my own closets as well. I was afraid of what was there, and it no longer seemed like a good idea to carelessly stir up the Kundalini pot to see what came running out. But I didn't want to live in fear either. Love and ecstasy training had illuminated some of my dark and dusty corners. Going forward, I wanted to be better prepared. I wondered what might be the natural predators of the scorpions hiding in the closets of my mind.

Chapter 15

Homeward Bound

The ache for home lives in all of us, the safe place where we can go as we are and not be questioned.
~ Maya Angelou

Yelapa was a cornerstone for our family. It was a time and place marked in the sand where we did something different, something unusual, something together. It was fodder for stories round the dinner table and college application essays. I grew up watching *Gilligan's Island* and dreaming of finding such a place. I mean, really, who gets to live for a time in a remote fishing village with no electricity, no cars, no phones, no TVs, no Internet, in a Swiss-family-Robinson-style palapa with hanging beds? Yelapa was my Gilligan's Island and it satisfied a deep itch within my being. It was not a final resting place, however. As idyllic as it seemed to be, there was always a part of us that could not fully relax. There was constant underlying worry: worry about the scorpions, worry about the kids staying well and safe, worry about having time alone together, worry about how we could contribute to this diverse community.

We realized that we were spoiled by the middle-class American way of life in which we were raised. One of the things about living in a remote place, for instance, was that getting the kind of medical help we were accustomed to was challenging. In the States, on the one hand, we were inclined toward natural and alternative healing, so we studied preventative medicine with some diligence, but on the other hand we did have a pediatrician we trusted to guide us through the ailments and medical predica-ments of young children. None of this was available to us in Yelapa. There was one medical clinic in town, but with the town drunk for a doctor, it was something of a joke. He rarely was at the clinic, preferring to drink heavily at the tourist beach.

About half way through our stay, Cassie started exhibiting strange symptoms. She wet the bed, for instance—something she had never done before—and craved sweet fruit drinks. She was normally a sweet, easy child, but began having wild mood swings. Also, large chunks of her back molars fell off. We began to get worried. We hiked up to the one phone in town and called our pediatrician back in the States, who suspected she might have pre-diabetes. There was no easy way for us to have her tested, but our pediatrician said we could take preventative steps. We were to keep her away from all sugar (so much for the independent walks down to the candy store) and to increase her protein intake. She was to drink water rather than fruit drinks as much as possible. This seemed to do the trick; she stopped wetting the bed and her moods calmed down. But it was an added worry for us.

Then, two months into our stay, we faced another medical emergency. Jake's parents had just left on the panga back to Puerto Vallarta after visiting us for a few days. Down near the launching beach, Jacki and her friend Bodhi were running up the trail to our casita together, while Cassie tagged after them, strug-gling to keep up. All of a sudden we heard a wail—not the kind you want to hear as a parent. Our little one had tripped on one of the pipes that crossed the path and her wrist had landed on the pipe. There was enough ruckus that some people came out to see what had happened. Jake and I ran over to her and could see that her wrist was injured. Jake picked her up and a woman motioned that we could bring Cassie into her little house to rest on the bed.

I was practically hyperventilating. She had gone from screaming to being suddenly, completely quiet and still.

Jake said, "Go. Run. Get the doctor!"

I ran over to the medical clinic and pounded on the door, but nobody was there. I called out to everyone, *"Dónde está el doctor?"* Someone indicated he was probably at the big beach, so I ran that way. It was a good 20 to 30-minute walk away along a very tricky path that climbed up and down the mountain, and over rubble and pipes. At one point, the path went through an abandoned building that had half collapsed from prior earthquakes. On the other side of the building, it passed through the silt river that changed every day, so you never knew how wide or how deep the channel would be. At the beach, out of breath and frantic, I yelled again, *"Dónde está el doctor?"*

Someone pointed him out to me, but I was more than a little distressed to see that he was actually totally drunk—slurring his words, unable to stand kind of drunk. I talked to him anyway, and because I was excited and fearful and couldn't remember how to speak, my words came out all mixed up, part English, part Spanish, part German. "My daughter . . . *Mi hija!*" I cried. *"Su manu está . . . kaput!"* I eventually got him to understand that my daughter had hurt her wrist. He looked back at me drunkenly and motioned out to sea, indicating I should try to get her on a panga and take her to Puerto Vallarta. But the last panga of the day would leave in about five minutes. I didn't have time. I turned and ran all the way back to town where Jake was still sitting with our girl. She had fallen asleep, thankfully. I explained the doctor was useless and that we had missed the last boat out. There was nothing to do but go back to our little casita and plan to take the first panga out to Puerto Vallarta in the morning. One of our friends heard what happened and came by our casita to tell us that by chance an English doctor had just arrived that day and that we could probably find him at his casita down the road a bit. We decided we would go look for him. He said he thought she had probably broken her wrist and agreed we should go to Puerto Vallarta first thing in the morning. Luckily, he had a mini-kit with him that included a sort of splint, which he wrapped around her wrist temporarily.

We slept fitfully that night, anxious to wake up early to make sure not to miss the panga. In the morning, we woke when it was still dark and scuttled around to get ready to go. Our attention for these brief moments was focused on the wellbeing of our daughter, and on getting everybody out the door . . . *not* on scorpions. In our hurry and worry, Jake had broken one of the golden rules and put his jacket on the ground. As we were racing about getting ready, he grabbed his jacket, slung it on, and felt something slide all the way down his back and land with a soft, but audible thud on the floor. He yelped loudly and we all turned to look. There at his feet was a large yellow scorpion — the biggest one we'd seen! He stomped on it quickly, but we all knew that we had let our "scorpion guard" down. It could have ended very badly.

We made it to the Puerto Vallarta hospital a couple of hours later. The x-rays confirmed that Cassie's wrist was broken in two places, so our little one got a shiny pink cast. As we headed back on the panga to Yelapa, we decided that it was time to make plans to go home, back to the United States. It wasn't just the lack of medical care, or the scorpions that called us home, although those were perhaps the proverbial last straw. We loved Yelapa, but we missed home, we missed family, we missed the United States, and surprisingly, we missed working.

It took us a week or so of hiking up to the one phone and fax in town every day to make the arrangements and get the necessary travel documents to fly back home. Our Yelapa experiment had come to a close. I loved the lifestyle of Yelapa. I loved the daily walking, the slow pace. I loved trading tie dyeing for food, and the sense of community I was beginning to feel with some of the folks there. But in the end, my life had other plans. There was work to be done.

After we returned to the States, I wrote in my journal:

Yelapa—what did it all mean? We could have scraped out a living by giving tantric workshops, tie-dyeing, eating cheap. But after a time, home called. Work called. We came to Yelapa looking to escape responsibility—to be gypsies. We left Yelapa to come home to hard work.

Yelapa gave me time and space to gear up for the real challenge that faced me. The challenge to face my fears, embrace my fears and let go of my fears—my tears.

I am Yelapa. There are scorpions in my closets.

(Journal entry, April 1997)

Part III

The Way

Chapter 16

Scorpion Eater Meditation

What you put your attention on grows.
~ Maharishi Sadashiva Isham (MSI)

L ife was a blur when we returned to the States. Jake almost immediately got a job offer to work for a start-up high technology company. It was a dream job for him, and he was happy to quit Boeing, from which he had taken a sabbatical. Boeing had become frustrating and bureaucratic, and although he had filed over half a dozen patents while at Boeing, he felt underappreciated and unchallenged. This new job opportunity was exciting and fun. I found my customers still had work for me and it was no problem to pick up my freelance paralegal business, but my real work was on myself.

Despite the great progress made in love and ecstasy training and the respite in Yelapa, I was still living in the shadow of fear, still crying every day. I wondered often, *What if I run into Shari in the grocery store? What am I going to do? How should I act?* But I was also afraid that I still didn't have a handle on who I was—that I couldn't nail down my identity. Was I happily married? Was I a good friend? A good mother? A good wife? A writer? Mostly, I sensed that my life was out of my control and I was afraid of having overwhelming feelings triggered. In other words, I was afraid my scorpions were just lying in wait to sting me and I wasn't sure what to do with them.

We had risked being vulnerable with each other by diving into our fears head-on. In the process we had revealed some hidden, dusty, scary corners. We recognized that we needed more tools to deal with our individual, as well as our relational issues.

I wondered, *How do I recover and fully heal from all the repressed scars of my early childhood? How do I keep my scorpions from unwittingly biting me? Most of all, how do I empower myself to rise above?*

Jake was still focused on the possibility of enlightenment. The timing was perfect when Jake came home one day, bearing an advertisement he had picked up. It read:

Ascension
Software for the soul

Learn powerful techniques to get in touch with the deepest part
of yourself
Relieve stress
Practice Praise, Love and Gratitude

Enlightenment guaranteed

"Look at this," he said with a funny smile. "They are claiming enlightenment is guaranteed! I think we should try it."

I perked up. The fact that Jake had any interest in such a flyer caught my attention; it seemed so out of character. Jake was an engineer by training. He liked facts. This was obviously an outrageous proclamation that was easy to prove wrong. But Jake seemed to approach it differently. If someone could be so bold as to *claim* that something as nebulous as enlightenment was guaranteed, well then, perhaps it was worthy of a second look. Some definitive experience must happen, he reasoned.

I thought about the trauma that had revealed itself during our year of love and ecstasy training. Instinctively, I felt that diving into meditation would help alleviate my PMS and PTSD symptoms; meditation might be the natural predator I was looking for, eradicating harmful thoughts and behavior. Perhaps

I didn't have to track down every last harmful thought, image, and stored memory through hours of therapy. Perhaps this was an approach that would allow them to dissolve more naturally. Thus began a new era in our life.

Ascension is a particular technique for meditating. It is not as well known as many of the more traditional meditation techniques, such as Zen or Vipassana (Mindfulness) or Qigong. It is related, however, to mantra technique, which many are familiar with because of Maharishi Mahesh Yogi's Transcendental Meditation™, which gained popularity in the 1960s and 1970s. The founder of Ascension and of the Society for Ascension (SFA) was Sadashiva Maharishi Ishaya, who had previously studied transcendental meditation, under Mahesh.

Ascension taught, at least initially, that no particular pose or position was required to be maintained while meditating. It was generally recommended that you keep your head higher than your feet, but even that was not required. The whole emphasis was on relaxing while meditating. You could even lie down if you wanted. At this stage, we were even advised not to worry if we fell asleep. In fact, it was stressed not to worry about anything, just do the practice, and keep doing the practice. The practice consisted simply of mentally saying an "Attitude," which was essentially a particular positive phrase, and then allowing that phrase to disappear without a trace. When it was gone, you would move on to the next one. There was a whole series of "Attitudes" to remember. If an unrelated thought came up, such as, *I wonder what is for dinner? Did I remember to give Jerry that book? What time is it?* you simply brought your attention back to the attitudes and said another one, allowing it, too, to dissolve. You continued until you had said all your attitudes, and then you started over.

Gently returning one's attention to the object of meditation, more commonly to something like the breath, is a tried and true method of meditation. What made this practice different and perhaps what contributed to its startlingly noticeable effect was that bit of brain candy thrown in. The brain had a little job. It had to remember these attitudes, these benign, positive sayings. Right away, I had fewer distracted, wandering thoughts when I started the practice, because my brain was slightly engaged in trying to remember the attitudes themselves. This was a marked difference from what happened the first time I tried a simple counting meditation at the Stonehouse Bookstore in Redmond.

The result was that very quickly both Jake and I could experience a more relaxed state and quieter minds than we had achieved on our own in Yelapa. I had fewer anxiety attacks, and our interactions with one another were less sticky. This was very encouraging and inspired us to keep practicing. We entered into the discipline of a regular practice together, which made it easier. Just as during our love and ecstasy training, entering into a commitment together gave us a shared goal—something new to focus on, something to practice together. We became a couple committed to growing together, instead of a couple struggling after difficult times.

What I didn't fully appreciate at the time, although I reaped the benefits, and which modern research has now proven with the advance of functional magnetic resonance imaging (MRI), is that meditation actually rewires the brain. For people like me, who suffer from unresolved childhood trauma, meditating bypasses the crippling "fight or flight" response, where the body begins responding as if it has been attacked: shaking and trembling, heart pounding, and uncomfortable hyper-vigilance and hyper-arousal.

Science has now measured and confirmed that meditation settles the amygdala's improper activation. A psychologist I met, Doug Brackmann, who teaches meditation to his clients, studied the recent scientific evidence on the effect of meditation on rewiring the brain. He explains in his classes, called "Zen, Buddha and the Brain," that the amygdala is like a primitive gatekeeper. Its job, he says, is to assess if there is a sudden change in the environment that is dangerous and then to compel a person to respond immediately without having to process the information. The problem, he explains, is that trauma can cause the brain to become miswired, so that the amygdala fires inappropriately, based on the memory of prior trauma, rather than anything currently happening. In such a case, even a harmless sound that mimics one that occurred during trauma, or even a thought of danger, can trigger an amygdala response that will generate PTSD symptoms.

He says we are wired to suffer. Luckily, meditation rewires the brain, not only by damping down the connections between the amygdala and the troubling thoughts, but also by increasing the neural connections that tie your cerebral cortex directly to your body and senses—essentially allowing you to be more present to what is happening in the moment, so that thoughts alone can't dump adrenaline into your body.

For me, what this meant was that by embarking on a serious meditation path, I was healing myself from my crippling PTSD response. Whatever had happened to me as a child or as an adult—the memories I had repressed—unresolved trauma—did not have to be unconsciously driving my behavior. Instead of repeatedly focusing on being broken, I focused on my techniques, which in turn reinforced different pathways, rewiring my brain to experience less fight or flight response and more peace, more stillness. And for Jake, he had a proven tool against his crippling depression.

* * *

Our "First Sphere Weekend" (the term that SFA gave to the introductory Ascension course) was hosted at a lovely house in Enumclaw with a gorgeous view of Mt Rainier out of the floor-to-ceiling picture windows of the living room. We gathered on a

Friday night and talked about what peak experiences we had had and what things were awe inspiring to us. Our instructor told us to choose a personal word or phrase that symbolized wonder or awe to us. We were cautioned not to pick something that carried any baggage with it, because our awe word would become part of the first Praise Attitude we were to learn.

It was an interesting exercise, choosing a word that captured my experience of awe. What inspired awe in me? *God?* I wondered idly. No, I decided. I had no personal connection with anything that I could refer to as God. The word really meant nothing to me, and there was plenty of baggage around the word. Beauty? Maybe, but it seemed sort of vague, as did Truth, and Love. I thought about Consciousness itself and finally settled on "Evolving Consciousness" — a mouthful, for sure, but something that made me feel hopeful and inspired.

The night after that first session, I developed a terrible headache. I literally felt like my head was being cleaved in two. In the morning, I could barely function, but we were determined to continue. I was pretty out of it during the lecture part of the session where we learned more about the mechanics of Ascension, but I took copious notes anyway.

What we learned is essentially what is reported on wikiedu-cator.org:

Ascension aims to reduce stress which has accumulated in the nervous system as a result of experience. It is believed that this stress becomes encoded into entrenched beliefs, behaviors and physical tension. Through Ascension, this accumulated stress is dissolved, resulting in expanded experiences of consciousness.

What I remember most, however, is that we were told we didn't have to try to understand our stress or the cause of it; all we had to do was allow it to arise and to bring our attention back to the process. This sounded like a simple way to eradicate scorpions to me, and ultimately it proved to be true; that is not to say, however, that the journey was *easy* or without suffering . . . thankfully, there were enough calling cards (namely, memorable synchronicities) and blissful experiences, even at that very first workshop, for it to be continually compelling.

Mid-morning, we learned the Gratitude Attitude, another phrase that fused the concept of gratitude with our awe word. After receiving it, we practiced meditating as a group for about 20 minutes. We were encouraged to be comfortable and to simply repeat the attitude over and over. If we noticed thoughts, we just came back to the attitude. I still had a terrible headache, but enjoyed the process well enough—nothing earth shaking. We took a break for lunch, then in the afternoon learned the Love Attitude and again gathered together to meditate as a group using that attitude.

Up to this point, I had enjoyed the workshop and thought everyone was nice. I was in prime "student" mode, however, eager to make sure I understood all the ins and outs and filling pages of my notebook with notes about everything the teacher said. He told us that over the course of our life we build up belief "grooves" that we are less than our infinite potential. He said Ascension cut through those grooves and got to the source, which they called the "Ascendant," where healing happens. He said Ascension decreases your heart rate. He mentioned all kinds of other wild statistics, such as 20 minutes of Ascension being akin to six hours of sleep, and that if you ascended three times a day for 20 minutes for one year, you would decrease your biological age by seven years. I wasn't really sure I believed what he was saying and was doubtful how the information had been gleaned. *Do they have scientific data?* I wondered. Still, I listened carefully and took notes. I liked the part where they said all I had to do was get out of the way, that I didn't have to try to under-stand my stress or the cause of it, that Ascension would dissolve any root stresses if I simply practiced it. I especially loved the lecture given before teaching the Love Attitude. Our teacher explained that the two root emotions are Love and Fear (False Evidence Appearing Real). Love, he said, was a choice to surrender control, attachment, judgment, and any ideas of victimhood. Ascension would help. I was reminded of my very first calling card, when the book *Love Is Letting Go of Fear* fell into my lap.

In the afternoon, we put our notebooks aside again and practiced the Love Attitude as a group. During that session I had an extraordinary experience. While ascending, I must have fallen asleep or something, although I recall being aware of the room. I imagined or dreamt that I was swimming in a warm ocean, but that my body was less dense than normal. It felt like there was space between the particles that made up the mass of my particular body. Those spaces or gaps became so enormous that diffusion with the surrounding environment was possible. I felt that I was commingling with the ocean as if my body had no boundaries, as if I was one with everything. It didn't last long—maybe a few minutes—but it was a breathtaking and memorable experience that captured my attention. I felt relaxed and happy at the end of the session; my heart felt unrestrained—open and free. My headache was completely gone. What had happened? Was I just imagining this? Was I experiencing existence from some completely different perspective? Was it a dream? Was that a normal experience from meditating? I didn't seek out the answers; I was content with the personal memory. Whatever had happened, it was new and different and if there was more of *that* available, I was all for it.

We quickly became hooked and almost immediately signed up to be sponsors. This meant that we could host events at our house and the teachers would come to stay with us. We thought this was an excellent idea, and a great way to meet more teachers. We became official "householders"—a term reserved for students

who were committed to meditating, but who also fully participate in a normal lifestyle, as opposed to living in a monastery or
ashram or convent. Our house became a meeting point for
ascenders, students and teachers alike. We loved being
surrounded by other folks who despite their own struggles had
made a commitment to search for more, to meditate regularly,
and to share with one another. It felt like there was something
greater going on and it was so much easier to calm the mind in a
group setting. Malika Chopra, Deepak Chopra's daughter, says
on that subject, "There is power in numbers, and there is no
power like a large group of people whose minds are attuned to
the same frequency of peace, compassion and joy."

Our fellow ascenders were all focused on praise, gratitude,
love, and compassion, and with each weekend retreat we
sponsored, our hearts opened a little more.

Committing to a regular practice of meditation and weekly
gathering with fellow meditators began to have a healing effect.
Essentially it allowed for a bit of separation from the problems of
our life that we thought defined us. It's not that we were
suddenly overwhelmingly peaceful, but rather that we began to
be aware that there was something quieter stirring within—a
space from which to witness our problems, instead of being
perpetually caught up in them. As the witness became more
prevalent, we began to realize that we were in fact more than our
thoughts, more than our social conditioning, more than our
conditioned reflexes, more than our pain. This is not to say that
meditating acts as an immediate panacea—in fact, often stuff
will bubble to the surface when you begin meditating, as if your
mind was just waiting for a quiet moment to remind you of all its
problems. While the discipline of meditation can be challenging,
because the mind will think of a thousand different reasons why
it is not a good idea to sit still, actually experiencing a quiet mind
is quite compelling. As our appreciation of that quieter space
within us grew, the pain of not committing to a regular

meditation practice was much greater than the challenge of doing it. We recognized, too, that it was easier to relax and trust the process if we surrounded ourselves as much as possible with people who were at the same stage as us, entertaining the same struggles (my back hurts, I'm bored, I don't have time . . .) and teachers who had been where we were now and could help us cut through any resistance.

Thus, over the course of the next year, we continued to seek out advanced retreats and to host weekly meetings and retreats at our house. We began to feel a sense of community with our fellow ascenders and some of the teachers. Here, at last, was a group of friends with whom we could grow.

In the fall, we met a group of ascenders for an advanced retreat being held in a ski lodge in the vicinity of Mt Rainier. It was a beautiful setting among an old-growth forest made up of western hemlock, Douglas fir and western red cedar. Nearby alpine meadows were still boasting late-blooming wildflowers. A dozen or so participants were present and a couple of teachers, one of whom we knew well. I noticed that she seemed a little withdrawn and approached her.

"Chandra, is everything okay?" I asked her quietly.

She paused, clearly deciding whether or not she should say something.

Finally, she said, "This is not public knowledge yet, but I just learned that the founder of Ascension, my Teacher, MSI . . . he's passed away . . ."

"Oh no. I am so sorry, Chandra. I had no idea!"

"It's okay. We have been expecting it. I am just going to miss him, but I am so glad that I get to be here meditating with you all."

All the teachers talked lovingly about the founder of the Society for Ascension, Maharishi Sadashiva Ishaya (MSI). We had hoped to meet him one day. He had even appeared to me in some sort of vision once when I had been meditating, and told me that the most important things were to drink water and not to give up.

Although the sad news threatened to make us gossipy from wanting to know more details, we all settled in a bit more deeply. I appreciated the focus of the group, especially of the teacher who had just received devastating news. That night at the group meditation, I felt the air grow thick and the room take on a surreal feeling. After sharing that silence, I noticed people spoke more deliberately and consciously. I felt "present," and suddenly knew what that meant, although I had heard it many times before. My mind was less distracted, less wandering. It seemed that my habitual thinking and worrying slowed and my focus narrowed to that which was occurring right at that moment. I felt keenly alive—magical—and sharing that effect with more people magnified it.

At first blush, we didn't think that MSI's passing would matter all that much to householders such as us. The organization seemed to be fully capable of functioning without him at the helm. Later, we would learn this wasn't exactly true.

* * *

After about six months of ascending, Jake became interested in Ascension's teacher training. He loved Ascension and believed it had tremendous potential to help not only himself on his quest for enlightenment, but also others. He believed the single most important thing one could do for the world was to become more conscious, and based on both of our heart-opening experiences with the ascension techniques, he believed this was the path to do it. He wanted to share it with the world.

The teacher training was offered at SFA headquarters in Waynesville, North Carolina. It was a six-month program that would require him to live on-site. As excited as I was to keep learning and practicing more, and as much as I understood and appreciated his interest in teacher training, it stirred up a lot of questions and feelings for me. What would that mean for our family? Our relationship? We talked about how we might do it — about the practical consequences of his going. Could we live on-site if I was participating as an assistant? Could we swap six-month programs so that he could go to one while I took care of the kids, then swap while I took the program and he took care of the kids? Once we graduated from the program, could we earn enough to support our family?

This was very different from the one-year love and ecstasy training. This would have a radical effect on our actual life circumstances that would include moving away from family, perhaps permanently, giving up our careers and committing to an entirely different lifestyle for both our kids and us. Frankly, I was not at all sure about the whole idea, but was willing to keep an open mind.

As we investigated a little more, we learned that there was a 17-day intensive prerequisite to teacher training. SFA offered two of these back-to-back in January and February immediately preceding the start of teacher training. We started to consider going to these.

In preparation and in order to be free from obligations, we actually sold our house to our neighbor, and then rented it back from him. This gave us a certain kind of freedom to explore different options and to be able to move, if we chose to. Meanwhile, I was doing a lot of research about the area, still trying to imagine how the whole scenario might pan out. Would we all move to North Carolina? Would the kids and I live in a town nearby while Jake went to teacher training? If so, what was the town like? What were the schools like? Could I get a job? I desperately wanted a sign or something to point me in the right direction.

One day, a strange thing happened that affected my decision. We came home from work and were getting ready to go out to a work-related holiday event later in the evening. I went to the computer to surf the net a little. I intended to learn more about the little town of Waynesville (outside of Asheville) where SFA was located. I pulled a search engine up (no Google yet) and started typing "Wayn—" when all of a sudden my computer screen went black. It stayed that way for a couple of seconds, then flashed unexpectedly to the home page for the Society for Ascension. It was not a page that I had bookmarked or anything, so it was a little startling. I glanced at it without much further thought, then went back to the basic search page and started to type in "Waynesville," but again, before I could even complete the word, my computer screen went completely black and then again came up on the SFA home page. It started to creep me out and I was wondering if SFA had some sort of cookies enabled or some sort of virus that directed your computer to their home page. I called a friend and fellow ascender and asked her while we were on the phone to go to her computer and repeat the steps I had just taken. Nothing happened for her. I hung up with my friend and then called Jake over to witness. I repeated all the steps with him watching over my shoulder and it did it again. He muttered something about that being weird, but said to leave it because we had to go to our party.

We went to the party that night, which was at a billiards hall in Seattle. The participants were all colleagues of Jake and were varying sorts of electrical and computer engineers. With this incident fresh in my head, I pestered all of them as to how my computer could have done such a thing. I explained exactly what had happened and what I had done and nobody had an explanation. They implied that I had imagined it.

We got home late that night, around 11:30 p.m. The computer was looming in the corner of our kitchen, beckoning me: "C'mon. Come see me. Try it again," it cajoled. I walked over, sat down, and took a deep breath, sure that the anomaly would be gone. I started typing into the search engine and sure enough the screen flashed black, then went to SFA's home page. I sat there dumbfounded until a curious thought crossed my mind: I wonder if there is something here I am supposed to read? I noticed then that there was a flashing entry that said "new." I clicked on it. The click took me to a memoriam for MSI, but my eye was immediately carried to the following words quoted from one of his books, which were displayed in italics in the middle of the page, and which have stuck with me ever since: "I come to you from beyond the portals of death, my beloved. We can never be sundered."

I didn't understand the mechanics or even the message necessarily, but it felt like an invisible hand from some realm other than this one had reached out and beckoned me personally to go deeper. I took it as a sign and made up my mind that we should go to the 17-day retreats. I knew what we had been experiencing in committing to a regular practice was tremendously powerful and reasoned it could only be a good thing to immerse ourselves more. We decided I would go to the first one in January 1998, and then Jake would go to the next one in February.

Chapter 17

Losing Control

Go into your fear. Silently enter it, so you can find its depth. And sometimes it happens that it is not very deep.
~ Osho

I was terrified. Seventeen days would be the longest that I had ever been away from Jake and the girls. Plus, over the years, I had become increasingly afraid of flying. It had come to the point where, despite my love of travel and desire to be a travel writer, I almost couldn't fly. The panic and terror I felt while flying did not trigger repressed memories per se, but the experience evoked the same physiological responses: hyper-vigilance, hyper-arousal, heart pounding. What was clear about flying was that I was not in control. As my fear grew, I depended more on Jake—burying my head in his arms and squeezing his hand in a death grip during takeoff. This would be my first time flying alone since developing that fear.

I began to have doubts about going and got serious cold feet the week before I was scheduled to leave. I worried about everything, starting with my fear of flying. I worried that I would have a panic attack on the plane. I worried about leaving the kids, about leaving Jake. But I also began to worry about SFA. Maybe it was a cult. Maybe this organization would strong-arm me into belonging once I got there, and I would get sucked into something that I couldn't get out of. All kinds of questions came up. What was this teacher training anyway? Why did you have to be sequestered and live on campus? Did we really want to abandon mainstream life again? What would be gained? Hadn't we been through enough already?

I decided to go to a hypnotherapist to see if I could shed some light on my worries and questions. I explained that I was afraid of flying and that I was worried about going on this retreat by myself. She approached the subject from the perspective that I must be afraid of dying and encouraged me to investigate that fear. But I couldn't relax during that session and we didn't get anywhere. She suggested that I continue to investigate on my own.

Back at home, I decided to delve into my fear of flying first. I knew it made logical sense that my fear of flying was tied to a fear of dying, but it just didn't feel right. I began ascending to get to a quiet space. Once I was relaxed, I intentionally imagined myself getting on the plane, finding a seat, and going through the takeoff. As I imagined all this, I could feel my body begin to react fearfully. With each imagined noise associated with takeoff, my body startled, and I became increasingly hyper-aroused and hyper-vigilant. I imagined looking out the window, studying the engines, looking for trouble. Even as I imagined the scenario, my heart was pounding. In my mind's eye I strained to look out the other side of the plane to check that engine as well.

Then, in a sudden insight, I saw it. I saw my fear. I wasn't afraid of my own death per se. Instead, I felt like I was responsible for the wellbeing of all the other people on the plane. I felt like I had to be in control and that it was up to me to listen for sounds that meant the engines weren't working properly. I needed to scan to make sure there were no fires in the engines. I needed to be the one to alert the pilot that the plane was in trouble. I felt responsible.

As this epiphany came to me, I had a sudden new realization: I was not the best person to be responsible for the safety of the passengers. I knew nothing about planes. I didn't know what was normal or not. I was ill-prepared to help. At the flight simulator in La Paz, Mexico, I had proven I was incapable of flying a plane. No wonder it filled me with so much anxiety. In a heartbeat, I saw that the pilots were in a much better position than me to take responsibility for the passengers. When I saw it for what it was, I was perfectly willing to turn the mantle over to the pilots. If I was going to fly, I was going to trust the trained professionals to take care of the plane and its passengers. It was as simple as that. That moment was 15 years ago. I have never been afraid of flying since.

Okay, so I could fly to North Carolina on my own. That left the issue of worrying about whether SFA was a cult. Finally, I called my mom and talked to her. I had a very close relationship with my mom and I trusted her. I told her just about everything. She had always been the kind of person you could go to when you had a big problem. She tended to hold back on advice, but when she gave it, you listened.

When I was a teenager, she didn't give the usual "don't drink and drive" talks or "don't have sex with boys" talk, but she did impress upon me to not get involved with any cults and to be very careful. Of course that was right around the era of the Moonies and Jonestown. I decided my mom would have good instincts and guide me right about going to the Society for Ascension. I anticipated she would talk me out of going, so I reached out.

"Mom, I am scared about going on this retreat."

"Why is that, honey?" she asked gently.

"Mom, what if they are a cult? What if they talk me into leaving my family?"

She paused for a moment and then said the greatest words you can ever hear from a mom.

"Honey," she said, "you are in charge and you get to make your own decisions. Nobody can make them for you. Relax. Enjoy. Go and check this organization out. It will be good to have some time to yourself. Don't worry about getting sucked into something stronger than yourself. You are strong. You will know what is right."

Strangely, just as I relinquished my hyper-responsibility and feeling that I needed to control life for everyone else, she reminded me that the only things I could control were my own discernment and decisions. And with that testimony, she handed me myself. She, the one who had seared the fear of cults into me in the first place, trusted me to do what was right. I felt better.

I also realized in some part of myself that if I really wanted to let go of my fear, I was going to have to dive in and really look at it. So in the end, the very fact that I was afraid to go made me realize I had to go. What was I really afraid of, anyway? Still, I wasn't completely ready to just sign up for the whole Society for Ascension, kit and caboodle. I decided to go, but as a way of hedging my bets I decided that I would go initially as an "observer." That way, I reasoned, I could see for myself what was going on. Was there some weird energy where people were being encouraged to leave their homes and families? Was there some underlying program beyond the simple benefits of meditating that I could discern? Would we be talked into drinking a strange Kool-Aid or covering ourselves in purple shrouds? I could be like a journalist. I could simply observe and take notes.

A few short days later, I found myself on a plane heading across the country. It was strange not having Jake at my side, but I knew that the only way to work out this longer retreat opportunity would be if we went separately, leaving the other at home to care for the children. As luck would have it, shortly after takeoff, a flight attendant approached me and said there was a spare seat in first class, would I like it? Absolutely! I settled back into my comfy chair and began to ascend. That flight was heavenly for me. I had none of the anxiety responses that I had always had while flying. I was relaxed and comfortable even though Jake wasn't there. As I ascended, both literally and meditatively, I felt completely at ease and peaceful. It seemed a very beautiful thing to be floating in the sky among the clouds. It was something like a miracle to me.

* * *

All I need is love . . . and a double tall non-fat latte.
~ Journal entry, 2006

It was snowing softly when I arrived at the Society for Ascension that January in 1998 still determined to be a journalistic observer. We were assigned bunks in the dormitory and shown the various buildings where different events happened. There was a main building with a large meeting room and dining area as well as several outlying homes nearby. We would meet in the morning in small groups at various teachers' houses nearby and again in the afternoon. I was pleased to learn that my group was to meet at MSI's house.

At night we were to gather in the main hall for what everyone called "the big meeting." Breakfast and dinner were served in the dining room at the main lodge. Our leaders recommended that we eat lightly to improve our meditations. The food was healthy and vegetarian. We were admonished not to drink coffee or eat chocolate.

The grounds were beautiful with walking trails through the woods to little secret gardens and ponds; there were giant rhodo-dendron trees everywhere and a spectacular main lodge with castle-like stone turrets and massive decks.

I kept to myself, refusing to engage in conversation or eye contact with anyone for the first 24 hours. As I am naturally gregarious and social, this was a strain for me. On the second day, I was in the communal bathroom when I inadvertently let down my guard and engaged in a light-hearted conversation with the woman standing next to me. Within a few moments, I was overcome with a rush of energy that traveled all the way through my body. I ran to the toilet and alternated between throwing up and having diarrhea. My whole body was shaking and I was incredibly weak. Someone ran to find a teacher; a woman all dressed in white, with long, cascading white hair walked in.

She knelt beside me with a gentle hand on my back and said, "Hi, I am Aramati. It's okay. I know exactly what is happening. You are a sensitive. You have just let the energy of this place into your body and your system is overcome. You are ungrounded. This happened to me, too. Don't worry, though, it will be okay, but you are going to have to eat meat, chocolate, and coffee, okay?"

I looked up into her beautiful and kind blue eyes and internally cracked up. Sure, I thought, here I am at a vegetarian meditation retreat where the only rules so far have been "don't eat chocolate or drink coffee," and my instructions are to break all the rules. As sick as I was, it made me relax, because I felt like I was being considered as an individual with unique needs. Maybe this wasn't a cult, plus who could argue with a mandatory sentence that required me to eat chocolate and drink coffee? This could be fun.

My fears were further alleviated one night, when one of the teachers, Durga, who was to become my best friend in later years, spoke up at the big meeting. In that meeting, we were encouraged to share whatever was going on with the whole group. A woman from Dallas stood up and said that she missed her family and wanted to go home. Other teachers in the room started to subtly shame her: "Don't give up." "This is important for you." "You need to stay." Then, Durga stood up and said, "She just told us she wants to go home, that she misses her family. She should go home and be with them, if that is what she has decided to do." My heart soared when she said that and my respect grew in leaps and bounds. Her forthrightness ended the discussion. Prior to that moment, I felt small, awed by what I perceived to be reverence in the air, awed by what I perceived to be great wisdom held by all the various teachers. When Durga spoke saying the opposite of everyone else, and standing up for the woman's own words, her own truth, I felt empowered. This was my journey. If I wanted to dive in, I could; if I wanted to go, I could. It was my choice.

I first met Durga in person when I was up at MSI's house for a group meeting. I lingered a little while after the meeting and was invited to join a group of teachers who were gathered in MSI's bedroom. Everyone was lounging about on the floor and on the bed when she came in, larger than life, somehow, carrying a big bowl of popcorn and laughing.

Her unruly, dark curls cascaded down her shoulders and her sparkling, big blue eyes lit up the room. She was dressed all in black and sporting a cast under her long black skirt. *She's beautiful,* I thought to myself, and my very next thought was that Jake would fall in love with her. I had heard she was MSI's girlfriend and that made her seem important in my mind—a goddess for sure. She was the center of attention in the room, charismatic, engaging, friendly. I wanted to reach for the popcorn just to have touched the same bowl.

I settled into the routine and found Aramati was right. If I ate a little heavier, I stayed grounded and my system did not rebel. That is not to say it was easy. Somehow, my visions of an extended meditation retreat included long hours of peaceful, blissful quiet. But when I started meditating in earnest, something else happened frequently—things seemed to get worse. All of a sudden as I practiced watching my thoughts, I became aware of all my negative thoughts. As I became aware of them I fought between two difficulties: one was to get swept up in those thoughts and to listen to their story again—not the goal of meditation; and the other was to desperately want those thoughts to go away and to try to will them away—also not the goal of meditation. It was a fine balance to allow thoughts and feelings to arise naturally and to let them drift away, all the while simply returning to the focus of meditation. Having the opportunity to practice this while on an extended retreat and to be encouraged to return simply to the focus of meditation again and again over days, even weeks, was invaluable. It's a bit like exercising. At some point you realize that if you keep at it—if you just follow the program—eventually it is going to get easier, but maybe not before you get really sore and tired.

Every morning at the retreat, I would get up and get ready for the morning session. I would actually primp for these sessions, as was my custom at home. Get up, get dressed, put on makeup, brush hair, look presentable, composed. With my makeup freshly applied I'd attend the first session and by mid-session all my mascara would be dripping down my face, since I invariably ended up in tears again and again and again as we were encouraged to share whatever we were going through. Someone would pass me a tissue, but I never really wanted the tissue, either. There was something about knowing that my composure was melting in front of all these witnesses that felt right. And sure enough, my scorpions willingly came scuttling out as soon as I settled down to ascend. On the outside, I had lived most of my life as a very successful individual. I had been voted "most likely to succeed" in high school and gone on to graduate summa cum laude from UCLA. I had started my own business, married a man I loved deeply and had kind-hearted, well-balanced children. I had been on wonderful and fulfilling adventures to exotic locales and was known for my cheerful demeanor. Even so, there were many different feelings combined with questions and worries that had been lurking inside me, driving part of my show, and contributing to traits like my excessive clinginess, which tended to come out at "certain times of the month."

I cried. A lot. I did note, however, that it wasn't always sadness bringing tears to my eyes—often it was gratitude. I was deeply thankful to be where I was, to have been afforded the opportunity to grow and change. At any rate, as one or another of us shared our stories, or as one teacher used to say: "the story of I," we would all listen and witness the sharing, then gently bring our attention back to the quiet, back to the stillness.

What I found interesting was that every day I would get up and do it again—carefully composing my outward appearance and applying makeup before going to the group session! I didn't even think to use waterproof mascara. I always started out looking like I knew exactly who I was and ended up looking like a disaster—but I didn't really mind. I recognized on some level that my mascara-streaked face was a more honest expression of my inner world. I didn't know anything. I was not composed.

I began to see a certain strength in my willingness to be vulnerable, to share my not-so-great stories, and to let others see that I was clueless. It was a whole new world I was exploring. I didn't have to know anything.

The extended meditation retreat allowed me the space to examine my inner world more closely and also offered me the opportunity to allow my negative thoughts and stuck feelings to pass on through. By and by, I started to get the hang of it: the thoughts would always be there, as would the difficult feelings. Meditation wasn't going to "get rid of them" as I had thought. Rather, meditation gave me the space to choose whether or not to focus on the stories or to rest in the gap between the stories.

My stories were tied up in my identities and things that had happened to me. I was a wife, a daughter, a mother, a paralegal. I had recently been betrayed by my best friends and had been traumatized as a child. But I wondered. Was that all I was? Was I my swirling, chaotic thoughts? Was the experience of my life, of living, constrained to roles that I played? Was the suffering I experienced all that was available to me? Who was I without my stories? What was lurking beneath the surface? Where did I get stuck? What programs were running unnoticed?

Despite my mascara-streaked face—my outward expression

of falling apart—I realized something else was happening, too. I was becoming curious. What was this part of me that could "witness" my thoughts? If I wasn't only the thinker, who was I? What was my pain all about? Was there some part of me that was inviolable, that could not be hurt? I became intrigued as to what part of my reactions and perceptions were conditioned responses. What did I really know to be true, anyway? Just because I thought something was bad, was it really bad? Was my experience of suffering a choice?

The retreat began to take on a different flavor. I realized for the first time that I needed to take the focus away from my relationship and back to myself. I needed to find who I was underneath my stories, underneath my perceived pain. I wrote in my journal:

> Pain is cultural baggage. One feels hurt because he/she has been conditioned to believe they are hurt. It takes courage to dive deeper than social conditioning to the truth of one's own heart . . . You can re-condition yourself to believe that you can't be hurt or you can go into your own heart and listen for the truth . . . The knowing inside must grow bigger. It must be more accessible. Does this tool I've been given work? Does it help? Try it for myself.
> (Journal entry, January 1998)

By the end of the 17-day retreat I was very relaxed. In fact, I was so relaxed I wasn't sure if I was ready to go home and dive back into my hectic life, even though I missed Jake and the kids. What would it be like? Would I be able to assimilate what I had learned? Would I be able to witness my thoughts back home? Would I be able to engage in my roles of wife, mother, daughter, and paralegal while maintaining some distance from them as well?

I also knew that as soon as I got home, Jake would be turning around and flying out here for his retreat, and he was coming with a mind to sign up for the teacher training. What would happen next?

Chapter 18

Householder or Seeker?

How does one establish an intimate bond without attachment?
~ Journal entry, 1998

"I'm coming home," Jake said.

"Really! It's a couple of days early; are you sure?"

"Yes. I am sure. I miss you guys and I want to be home for Valentine's Day."

Jake had just completed 14 days of his 17-day retreat. While he had expected to be signing up for the six-month teacher-training course at the end of the retreat, he discovered that he didn't want to do the teacher training. He wanted to come home early and be with his family. Some moments are so precious.

We also learned that SFA was starting a new program to support householders such as ourselves. They were opening satellite centers in various areas that would offer on-site teachers and weekly ongoing meetings as well as regular local retreats. A satellite office was to be opened in our city! And Durga was to be one of the teachers living at our satellite center. Now it seemed possible to keep exploring our inner world, to rest in the stillness of the ascendant, and to continue fully participating in our lives as householders. We were excited.

There was the issue of our house, which we had sold, but now that the direction of our life was not so uncertain, we decided to buy another house in the area. Jake, still susceptible to seasonal affective disorder from the multitude of gray days in Washington

State, decided that he wanted a house with lots of light and a big view.

We settled into our beautiful new house, perched on the edge of Somerset Hill, and watched the seasons change. The view was magnanimous and magnificent, affording sunsets all year round. We created a private hot-tub area we called the "jasmine courtyard," lined with lacy bamboo and sweet-smelling shrubs. From here we could comfortably soak outside during all the wet and drizzly Seattle days. As we enjoyed the material fruits of our labors, I still noted how difficult it was to integrate my inner and outer worlds, and difficult to divide my time.

There was still work to do. I wrote:

The creation here in our new home is paradise, yet still it is our inner houses we work on—we struggle with. One day building a courtyard of hope inside, the next collapsing from despair.

These homes, our inner and outer, both need attention and maintenance . . . I search for the path that nurtures my soul, that frees my spirit—that maintains my inner sanctum even as I toil to maintain my outer home.

(Journal entry, spring 2000)

And my inner home still troubled me. The despair I wrote about in my journal would come over me like a wildfire, reigniting all my old worries—many of them still about Shari. *What if I run into her? Will I be able to be calm and centered? Or will my heart beat wildly out of control?* Just imagining the scenario made my heart beat faster, panic rising in fear of what my reaction might be. I knew I still had work to do.

As my commitment to the nurturing of both my inner and outer houses grew, I quickly became attached to both. I could not see the difference. It seemed to me that I made a commitment because I appreciated the value of something: being married to

Jake, having a family, meditating regularly, for instance. Once I appreciated the value of something, I couldn't imagine life without it, which triggered my worrying about losing it: the very crux of suffering. In fact, I had created a perfect maelstrom for suffering by being attached to two very different paths—that of the householder and that of the seeker.

It would be many years before I appreciated the difference between commitment and attachment, but the seeds were planted during this era when I began to ask my own questions and to inquire more deeply into the nature of intimacy and attachment, deeper into fear and surrender. It felt like time to move again into uncharted territory. *What boundaries am I attached to? Which ones can yet be removed? How much more can I surrender? Which of my habitual and conditioned responses no longer serve me? What do I need to let go of to grow further?*

Chapter 19

A Sexual Road Less Traveled

But Rumi is not satisfied with little miracles. So the party gets cranked up more as he keeps dancing, and all of a sudden the *wagon master* shouts,

When I am done with you, the firmament will be smeared all over your face; even your asshole will be a shrine.

And some hearing such ribald language sing back,

Thank God! Thank God! Hallelujah baby, someone just told me the truth.

But then a few others walk away, thinking,

Blasphemy, how could every part of me be holy?

What to say? It has been long known: good poetry is also meant for the high rollers in the barroom where the talk gets gritty and real—as well as for the pious in the mosque, temple, and church.

~ From the introduction, titled: The Wing Comes Alive in His Presence, in the Penguin publication *The Purity of Desire: 100 Poems of Rumi*, by Daniel Ladinsky

Sex. No question—it is fertile ground for growth, fertile ground for uncharted territory. Our foundation in love and ecstasy training, and relief from prior sexual trauma through regular pelvic release sessions, combined with our newly acquired base in quietness and witnessing through Ascension meditation practice, allowed Jake and me to explore any remaining unplumbed depths. We developed a habit of scheduling lunch dates during the workweek where we met back at home, while the kids were in school, to explore and play with each other. This gave us the time and space to slow down our lovemaking as we had been trained to do—to pay attention to what was going on inside—and to push or at least investigate the nature of boundaries that may have been limiting our experience.

We'd prepare a sacred space and our bodies, brushing our teeth, cleaning our nether region, bringing ourselves to the bedroom clean and ready.

Taking a few breaths, I repeat a couple of attitudes, my form of meditation, which brings me back to the moment as a player and witness combined. I notice the layers of pride mixed with self-judgment I carry with me. When one or the other reigns, I have lost myself, lost the moment. But there are times when the moment is so full that "I" am lost in another way altogether. A feeling of timelessness sweeps forth ebbing and flowing. I begin to touch him.

It took years for me to understand massaging another is as much a gift to oneself as to another. When one fully gives and the other fully receives, wholeness is reached.

I feel the subtle energy flowing through me to my hands and to him. The connection meets the moment. The passage of time is marked vaguely by the physical sensation of tiring as time passes or of music stopping or of awareness that enough time has been spent in one place.

I take my time now as I reach the buttocks and play with the sacral joint—with the entrance to the anus. "A little softer" he whispers. "Ah yes. That feels good." I penetrate the opening of his darkest hole—you wouldn't want to go there, the "good" parts once said. Now I let my tongue wander to the opening as well. Why not? He sighs pleasurably, gently releasing tension. Why not? I probe deeper. Is it bad? Where have these rules come from? I fear breaking the rules—but now I've broken so many and experienced so much more than

I might have. We need rules! All those "good girl" parts of me scream. They keep order. But do they enliven me, awaken me, free me, a new part of me inquires?

I ask him what it was like. He tells me it was relaxing, pleasurable, that as taboo as it seems, the area is very sensitive—as sensitive as the lingam [penis]. He says it helps him imagine what it must be like for a woman to be pleasured.

(Journal entry, 1999)

The experimenting went both ways as we became curious as to what the boundaries were, if any. I became curious about surrender—what did that look and feel like? Having exposed my scorpions, I wasn't so afraid of what might be lurking in my mind. I trusted the process of being vulnerable and was willing to experience beyond the gateways of my mind. We knew how to communicate clearly, how to respect each other, how to trust that even pain and taboo might be a doorway to more.

With our new foundation and a growing experience of staying centered, I found I wanted to explore the broader concepts of aggression versus submission, of devotion and surrender in our sexual practices. I was curious about whether I could get beyond the fortress of my fear, held tightly by my mind.

I discovered that when I felt connected, when the air felt still, when I approached certain sexual practices with devotion, the experience took on a new dimension beyond the simple acts. I found that when I let go of fear, love flew in.

The Sexual Road Less Traveled

What is that unexpected rush
That sends my body into
Ecstatic expectation?

As my nipples harden, I realize with some surprise,
That they are eagerly anticipating being squeezed.
My mind balks at their response, yet it is undeniable.
Body does not always follow mind, I think.
Sometimes, body responds to a deeper wisdom.

The body knows,
That within the sharp piercing pain
Of nipples being squeezed hard,
Or of buttocks being whipped
There is
Sweetness,
Stillness.

Within the Yang
Of aggression
Is Yin.

I move closer to him, allowing the rest of my body comfort I invite
him to
Squeeze my nipples.

Does he know, I wonder
That it feels as if my nipples are pincushions,
And that he is sticking them with pins?

I watch him.
What I see reflected is
Innocent joy.

I am That.
I realize

How could I know it could be so?

For in his rush to pinch, my mind panics,
And becomes too quickly
An impenetrable fortress,
Unwilling to let down its guard.

But, fortunately curiosity creeps in,
And I wonder if the pain is really all there is.
"Take me with you,"
I beg.

"Take me on that journey before my mind has held fast."
He releases and starts again.
This time I hold my mind in the cradle of my heart and Surrender
to a greater truth.

I relax.

I feel the pain, but, I note, I find it exciting not fearful.
I feel like I'm flying.
Ahhhhh such sweet surrender.

This, I realize, is what my body too yearns for.

"Do it again," I beg,
And together, laughing at the absurdity,
We travel a sexual road less traveled.
(Journal entry, 1999)

Chapter 20

Parenting on the Path

Question: What is the meaning of life?
Answer: God is everywhere.
~ Jacki, our nine-year-old daughter

Despite our less traditional path, life was busy in all the normal "householder" ways too, from holding down jobs and raising our children to participating in all the fun activities of parenthood, such as swim lessons, girl scouts, bike riding, camping, arts and crafts, trips to Grandma and Grandpa's, and volunteering at school; it's just that it was also peppered with mini Ascension retreats and regular daily ascending—two or three 20-minute sessions per day as we endeavored to meld our two lives. Our own experiences on the path thus far had shown us that life was not all it seemed to be at first glance and this affected our parenting. We listened to our kids differently, not as quick to shun or disbelieve—not so sure that we knew the "correct" answer. We told our kids all the time to investigate what was true for themselves.

Like many other parents, however, we wanted to share our spiritual leanings with our kids. We offered them each the opportunity to learn to ascend if they wanted, although we left the decision up to them. Jacki, who was nine years old by this time, was not really interested. Perhaps this was because she was simply more evolved than we were. As we struggled to search for the truth, it was already obvious to her. I found a crumpled-up, folded piece of paper in her room one day around this time—

the kind that kids make where you pick a number, which refers to a question, and then unfold a flap to find the answer to the question. I read the question: "What is the meaning of life?" and then unfolded it to read: "God is everywhere."

But we also knew she was a little wary about Ascension since it had almost led to her father spending six months away from her for teacher training. One day before we went on our 17-day retreats, I volunteered in her third-grade classroom. After helping the kids write their own delightful version of "Desiderata," the poem by Max Ehrmann, I walked down the hall on my way to the car. It was just before Christmas and Jacki's teacher had posted her students' letters to Santa on the walls. I paused and read a few: "Dear Santa, please bring me a Pokémon Gameboy for Christmas"; "Dear Santa, I would like a new Beanie Baby and a Tamagotchi for Christmas." I scanned the wall looking for my daughter's letter, curious to see what she wanted for Christmas. When I found it, the hallway suddenly got very long and narrow; my heart simultaneously plummeted and soared. She had written: "Dear Santa, please bring my daddy enlightenment for Christmas so he won't move to North Carolina." We didn't question Jacki about what she had written, since she hadn't said it to us. Rather we allowed her words to simply take hold of our hearts, lest on our quest for more we missed what was right in front of our face. We had learned that even parenting was less about telling and more about listening.

While Jacki was tentative about Ascension, Cassie was decisive and told us she did want to learn. A highly sensitive girl with a bright, dimpled smile, she has surprised us on more than one occasion with her eerie premonitions and other phenomena. She regularly pulled exact words out of my mouth before I spoke them and had her own regular contact with the world of spirits.

When Cassie was five, I went to tuck her in one night and heard her looking at the ceiling and counting. She was concentrating.

"One, two three, four . . . "

"What are you counting, honey?"

"I am counting the spirits, Mommy. But shhhhhhh. They are shy and they will go away easily."

The spirits?

"What spirits, honey?"

"The good white ones, Mommy."

"White ones?"

"Yes, Mommy. There are white ones and black ones. The white ones are nice, but the bad ones are black. Everyone has some. You can see them hanging around people. Oh, see now, they went away. They don't like us talking about them."

I had no idea what to say to this, so I just nodded. This lasted until she was about nine or ten and then she stopped doing it and would get embarrassed if we asked.

She loved ascending, however, and would do it every night before she went to bed. She said it helped her sleep and made her dreams better. She was very innocent about it and would change her special awe word all the time. It might be "dolphins" or "teddy" or "sunshine" on any given day. One day, she and I got in a fight about crepes. She wanted crepes and I told her she had to wait, for some reason or another. She stomped her foot and got very upset. I suggested she calm down and asked her if she wanted to ascend for a few minutes with me.

"Oh, okay," she said.

"Do you have a special word?" I asked.

"Yes," she said. "It's going to be crepes!"

In her world, in that moment, the most awe-inspiring thing was a serving of crepes. It cracked me up.

During this era, I had the opportunity to volunteer in her first-grade classroom and I believe the momentum of regularly ascending helped me to be more playful and opened up a space to be creative and light-hearted. I didn't feel as constrained by what was appropriate or proper and was not worried about how

I appeared to other adults. Cassie's classroom needed an art and science docent and I decided to do both. The teacher told me that they were working on an insect unit and perhaps I could work around that. I thought it would be fun to do it in a way that had never been done before.

On the first day of my docent duty, I arrived at school in costume. I was dressed up in a bright yellow hazard suit with a pink neon radiation sign on the back. I wore large antennae and garish hot-pink wing-tip sunglasses. I came into the classroom and announced solemnly that I was Dr Zorg from Inner Space and that I was here to study the Planet Earth. My mission was to study interesting bugs and bring back vivid drawings and reports. I had heard that children were great observers and that the best way to learn was with children. Would they be interested in entering into this mission with me?

"Yes!" they all chorused.

"Great!" I said. "Now the only other thing you need to know is that people from Inner Space can't tolerate a lot of unruly noise, so if it gets too noisy or rambunctious in here, I will have to retreat to Inner Space for a while."

"Okay . . ." they said, not sure what to make of me.

I explained that I was going to work one-on-one with each of them to create a drawing and report about an insect of their choice. Then each of them would have the chance to share their drawing and what they had learned about their bugs with the class.

It was a wonderful experiment. I would come each week with a large picture book that had great drawings of insects that we could copy and work with one of the children. Each child would pick a different insect that interested him or her and then make a giant poster-size colorful drawing. While they were working on the drawing, I would look up facts about that particular insect and the child would select the ones that interested them. The insects they picked were fantastic, and I loved learning along with them about the rhinoceros beetle, which could carry more than 100 times its own weight, or the blue morpho butterfly, whose lifespan is only 115 days, or the monarch butterfly which migrates twice a year for close to 3000 miles.

At the start of the next week, I would stand up in front of the classroom (in my Dr Zorg outfit) and introduce the child that was going to come up and share their drawing and the favorite things they had learned about their insect. Sometimes, when I first arrived the class was noisy and a little rambunctious, excited for the session. When that happened, I would suddenly stop talking altogether, close my eyes and put my arms to my sides, hands in classic mudra position (index fingers to thumbs, other fingers outstretched)—a symbol that I had had to retreat to Inner Space because it was too noisy in the classroom. In short order, a hush would fall over the room and we would begin again. The session became so popular that the teacher invited the other first-grade classroom to participate as well.

Also during this time, a fellow ascender and I decided that we wanted to volunteer at a local hospital. We wanted it to be light-hearted and fresh, and our idea was to just sit with people or maybe to bring in some gifts. We dressed up in skirts and wore angel wings and then headed to one of the wards, where we wandered around looking for people who looked alone and lonely. We would ask permission to come into their room and then sit with them and just talk. My friend was a massage therapist, so she would hold their hand and rub it gently, or ask them if they would like some of the various scented, natural-essence lotions she had brought along. I would sometimes bring along a bagful of silk scarves I had picked up at a thrift store and offer them up, draping them around necks or hanging them up in the room for a spot of color. The patients loved it. They would tell stories to us or express their gratitude. Sometimes they cried. The nurses loved it too. They said their patients always did better on the days we came. Unfortunately, we had not followed strict protocol in setting up these volunteer visits and eventually, we were told we either had to go through human resources to officially set up a program or could no longer come. We decided not to create a more formal program. It had been time well spent, but its time was done.

In so many ways, life was juicy and very good. I was freed up to be more spontaneous and creative in ways I never would have considered before, both in my public and private lives. I wondered, though, what it would take to really let go of all my fear. What does it take to fully surrender? *Maybe,* I thought, *I can unburden the fortress of my mind from its emotional pain as well.*

My heart was opening and it made me realize I still wanted more. What I didn't fully appreciate at the time is that getting to "more" was not necessarily a jaunt down Easy Street. It would require the willingness to enter what some call "a dark night of the soul."

Chapter 21

Settling the Muddy Water

Muddy water, let stand—becomes clear.

~ Lao Tzu

Despite the sweetness and light-hearted endeavors in my life at this time, a nagging thought kept pestering me. Even though it had been five years since I walked in on Jake and Shari, and even though Jake and I had done significant healing work together and traveled down uncharted intimate roads since that time, I hadn't completely forgiven *her*. Plus . . . I had the nagging feeling that forgiving her was not really enough: I needed to thank her. I felt deep within myself, in a corner where I wasn't willing to look very often, that even though I was struggling and sometimes near despair, I was also eternally grateful to have been afforded the catalyst to action—the catalyst that revealed repressed memories, memories that had previously conditioned my responses to life—the catalyst that encouraged me to look inside the deep, dark corners of my mind to expose the negative thoughts for the scorpions they were—the catalyst that encouraged me to take a risk and be vulnerable, that allowed me to be more alive and less afraid. Shari, however inadvertently, precipitated my journey. I knew someday I would call her. I also knew it could not be rushed. So, I periodically checked in with myself. *Are you ready to call Shari? To forgive her? To express gratitude?* I would silently ask myself. No. Not yet.

The nagging thought began to get more urgent. There was a battle happening in my heart. *Are you ready yet?* No. Not yet. I can't do it yet. *Okay.* Then some weeks or months later, *How about now?* NO, I CAN'T! She hurt me. She betrayed me. Why should I forgive her? And the silence in my heart would wait patiently. *No problem. Just checking.*

As this battle ensued inside me, I became increasingly agitated, and despite our regular meditation practice and support, I began experiencing panic attacks again. I still worried I was going to run into Shari and that terrified me. She began creeping into my dreams. She'd show up in the periphery—a glance of her at a party or something. Then the dreams became more insistent and she showed up front and center. One night I dreamed the affair had led to a pregnancy and I woke up in terror and filled with raging jealousy. Despite my training, I didn't talk to Jake about these dreams. I was too embarrassed and scared. It felt like there was a knot inside that needed to unravel but was not quite willing. I was afraid to let go of something that had become a part of me—my hurt at having been betrayed by her. I felt righteous about my feelings—they were deserved, right? Everybody would agree. But as I went deeper into myself, entertaining the possibility that those feelings were no longer serving me, I felt a kind of despair at letting them go, and I desperately wanted someone else to do the work; I wanted Jake to bail me out. Instead, as the energy built, I got into more fights with him. I approached my first dark night of the soul—a period of time marked by a cloud of unknowing—a time of agony, suffering, pain, and unusual physical sensations.

I don't know why the downward cycle happened, but I came to learn it is not unusual on a spiritual journey. At certain junctures, some part of oneself wants to cling to everything it once knew to be true—even if those things do not serve one. A teacher once explained that sometimes before a leap in consciousness, you have to fall back to get a running start. At any rate, the feelings were overwhelming. Even so, there was an honesty to them. They were raw and pure. Despite my resistance,

I knew on some level that the only way out was to actually experience the physical and emotional feelings. In my diary I wrote:

> I cry that nothing is as simple as it was . . . I seem stuck in some nightmare of feelings that threaten to overcome me . . . All I can do is feel and be depressed. I'm dying. I want joie de vivre and instead what I have is a heavy heart, a heavy soul . . . part of me knows that if this is not true, nothing is. Have I lost all perspective? Why does it seem so big? It seems like everything is at stake. I long for sweet words. Nothing but sweet words . . . My life is a roller coaster despite all attempts to find peace and calm within. I believe in nothing. Perhaps that's the heart of the problem—I don't know what to believe in . . . Depression scares me. It takes so much light out. It is so cloying, so seductive. It seems to take more than I have to crawl back out.
> (Journal entry, 28 February 1999)

These dark writings scared me, but at the same time engendered compassion for myself. I learned to focus on the actual physical sensations instead of the thoughts and began to appreciate the part of myself that was willing to feel. My very next entry less than a month later reads:

> My own words shock me with their impact. I read my last entry and I feel for that self, for that moment . . . I've been experiencing this feeling in my chest for the last couple of weeks, a kind of tingling rush, a current. It's an underlying feeling, ever present and gets stronger when I meditate. I can feel it now, if I focus. It's as if a part of me is a flowing river, or perhaps a waveguide, a channel electrified by the current passing through. I feel it in my belly and legs too, less in my throat and head, but somewhat present there too.

I rant. I rave. I cry. Mostly I cry, wanting to be heard, to be received. Is mine a tormented soul? I would never think so, but reading my diary that's what you'd sense. The cheerful moments are less likely to inspire me to write. It is always my darker days that bring pen and paper together . . . I am not a tormented soul. I don't see myself that way—only an open channel for much energy to flow through. More and more I experience my body as a conduit through which life's energy flows. My nervous system is a powerful communicator because I am willing to feel too much.
(Journal entry, 9 March 1999)

I didn't realize it at the time, but these were also classic signs of Kundalini rising: surges of vibrating energy in the body, uncontrollable weeping spells, outbursts of temper, feelings of great neediness, clinging to others, sudden episodes of anxiety, fear, rage, grief, guilt, depression, despair, hopelessness, exaggerated fears, deluge of memories of events from the past. To me, it felt like a massive maelstrom of negativity.

I longed for Jake to wrap me up in his arms and whisper sweet words in my ear—something he was prone to do, except when he wasn't, which usually happened when I was extra needy. As the nagging thought grew in the back of my mind that it was time to let go of my hurt, so did a desire for external proof that I was lovable, that I was worthy. I clung to Jake. As my neediness grew, Jake's inclination to comfort me diminished. It was a vicious cycle.

It culminated one night when I grew so upset I did not sleep all night. I tried to get Jake to talk to me, to comfort me, but he was frustrated with my intense moodiness, and just rolled over and went to sleep. I got up, broken-hearted, and left the room—heading I didn't know where. I ended up in the basement, huddled on the floor in classic child's pose, bent over and hugging my knees, naked and cold, but not caring, only feeling sorry for myself—feeling alone and separate, thoughts of despair circling. I wailed into the dark cold night, deep, gut-wrenching, heart-wrenching sobs. I hate this. I hate life. What's wrong with me?

Some part of me felt like it was time—time to let go, time to call Shari—but I simply could not stomach the thought. What confused me most was that I had believed our friendship was deep and lasting. I couldn't reconcile that with her behavior. My general thoughts of despair turned into specific thoughts about my friendship with Shari. Had she never really liked me? Had I done something to her? Had she always just had a thing for Jake? *If I do call her one day,* I agonized, *what will she say? How will she respond to my call? Does she hate me? Do I hate her? Will we just have a screaming match?*

I was shivering uncontrollably now. I crept upstairs and found an old hooded sweatshirt in the closet that I pulled on over my head. My address and phone book caught my eye and I reached over and scrolled through the listings. There was her number. Without thinking about it, I copied it down on a ripped scrap of paper and stuffed it deep into the pocket of the sweatshirt. I wandered back into the living room and sat numbly waiting for dawn.

In the morning I was weak and overwrought but managed to get the children to school. Once the children were off, I paced around the house, like a tiger stalking its prey—except it felt more like I was the prey and a tiger was stalking me. I couldn't breathe, I couldn't think. I didn't know how to move forward. Every noise caught my attention, as if my demise was imminent. Finally, I grabbed my cell phone and keys and ran out of the house, literally in flight, away from . . . something. I had no destination in mind, so I drove aimlessly around the neighborhood, not knowing where to go or who to talk to.

I landed in the parking lot of Loehmann's department store, about a mile from my house. I stopped the car and sat staring at the dark, wet pavement in front of my car; all around shoppers were busy going about their business, but my world was small. I stared out my front window through my own teardrops at the raindrops gathering on the pane, feeling separate from everyone and from life.

Finally, I called my mom. "Mom," I sobbed into the phone.

"What is it, honey?" she said, sounding concerned.

"Mom, I need help! I don't know what to do! I can't go on . . . "

Mom, who had certainly heard me in all manner of upset before, must have heard something different in my voice that day. She got quiet and decisive at once. Calmly she told me, "Honey, I can talk to you of course, but I think maybe you should hang up with me and call the crisis hotline. They will know what to do and say. Wait one minute and I will look up their number."

She came back and read the number to me. I reached into my sweatshirt pocket and found a crumpled piece of paper in it and an old pen in the car. I scratched the number for the crisis hotline on the paper. My mom made me promise I would call the crisis hotline and that I would call her back in one hour.

I hung up with my mom and sat in the car, fingering the paper. Then I noticed it was the scrap of paper on which I had written Shari's number. I paused. Call Shari or call the crisis hotline. Call Shari or call the crisis hotline. I wanted to call Shari, but I couldn't do it.

I dialed the number for the hotline, heart pounding, ready to pour my guts out to a stranger—to someone trained to help me— someone to make me feel better—but I was greeted with a busy signal. What? How could the crisis hotline be busy? Wasn't that their claim to fame—that they were there at all moments to talk people off the ledge? I hung up and tried again—still busy.

Suddenly, I found myself laughing out loud. All the accumulated stress and worry and gut-wrenching despair evaporated. The circumstance clearly was a cosmic joke—or perhaps another breadcrumb in life? No one was available to help me: not Jake, not my mom, and not the crisis hotline—life was pointing me to a different solution. I was going to have to rely on myself and, really, I knew exactly what to do. I picked up the phone and dialed the other number.

"Shari?"

* * *

I walked under the covered front porch of the cozy, light-blue, two-story country home out in Maple Valley. It was a comforting place, with lots of kitsch floral décor and overstuffed furniture. Out back, donkeys brayed, rabbits hid in the corners of their hutches, and chickens scuttled about. The aroma of coffee filled the air.

Depending on the time of year when I visited, the abundant vine maples lining the street in front of the house would lend either a vibrant green or a splash of orange and red underneath and amid the dark Douglas firs. Today, I appreciated the bright yellowish-green color of the spring leaves.

This was the home of my hairdresser, Diane, and I loved coming here. She and her husband were transplants from Los Angeles, where once upon a time they had done hair for celebrities. They tired of the hustle and bustle and moved to a quiet corner of Washington State to live out their dream of a ranch house in the country. She had built a little hair studio into her house, right off the kitchen and family room with a view to her backyard. Her husband retired from the hairstyling business to take care of their little ranch, but if we clients were lucky, he offered to help her out by washing our hair; he gave a wonderful head massage. Diane never advertised; you had to discover her by word of mouth and I was lucky to have found her.

The trek out to her house took about 45 minutes, plus she was always running late. Part of the experience was sipping coffee in her kitchen with her other clients while you waited for your turn. Generally the outing took the whole morning or afternoon. When the kids were little and not in school, it was great, because she had a big family room with an enormous television where they could sit and watch Disney shows while I got my hair done. I had shared her as a resource with my friend Shari, and Diane quickly became Shari's hairdresser too. Often, we would try to coordinate our visits, so that all our kids could play together and we could totally relax at our own version of a country day spa.

After the initial split with Greg and Shari, I used to worry about running into Shari at Diane's house. But five years had passed without ever running into her. When our ex-friends moved to Bainbridge Island, I was sure Shari wouldn't travel an hour and half to get to Diane's, so I stopped fretting about it.

It was an odd surprise, then, to walk into the house and run into Shari, who was just leaving. It could have been really awful, but this chance encounter happened less than a week after I had called her on the phone. We had already made our peace with each other.

The day I had called—the crisis hotline day—I had at last reached the point where I was ready to forgive her and, in fact, to thank her. I knew exactly what I wanted to say and I planned to say it quickly before she could say anything angry or upsetting that would change my mind. When I called her that day and said her name, she immediately recognized my voice and began crying and talking urgently.

"Mariah! I am so sorry for everything that happened. I didn't want to call you because I didn't think you would ever want to speak to me again. But since you called me, I want you to know you were the best friend ever. I had no right to do what I did. It was selfish and stupid and I lost so much. You did nothing wrong. I had my own demons I was wrestling. I have no excuse, I know, I just want you to know I am so sorry . . . "

Although I had come to the point where I no longer needed to hear them, her words were an unexpected salve to my soul.

"Shari . . . you have no idea how nice it is to hear you say that. I've been wondering, stressing over whether I imagined our whole friendship, which I greatly appreciated at the time. So thank you for your kind words. But actually there is something I want to say." I paused, gathering my strength. "So much has happened in the last years. I want you to know, first, I forgive you."

She murmured a sweet noise of gratitude. I took a breath and went on.

"But it's more than that. In many ways I am actually . . . well . . . grateful for what happened. It has been a powerful catalyst in my life and has given me an opportunity to examine dark corners of my own self that I barely knew existed. It has forced me to grow and to search for deeper meaning in life. So, thank you, for your role. Maybe it was meant to be."

"Oh, Mariah," she responded, "I'm so glad to hear that. I've just felt so horrible . . . " She trailed off.

As the conversation came to a close, we kept it honest and didn't promise to become friends again or even to see each other, but there was a feeling of honoring what had once been and an acceptance of its completion. On some level, I could see that she and I were just imperfect beings doing the best we could with what we had been dealt. I recalled then that her mother had committed suicide when she was about four years old, and I wondered what effect that might have had on me if the situations had been reversed.

So when I ran into Shari that day at Diane's, I was not incapacitated by a panic attack, as I had feared. I was calm, and we exchanged easy pleasantries and marveled for a minute how glad we both were that we had happened to talk prior to running into each other. She, too, had feared a chance encounter.

"Guess what?" I told Jake when I got home. "I ran into Shari at Diane's today."

"Wow! How did that go?" he asked.

"It was fine. Sounds like the kids are doing well. She, Greg and the kids moved and live on one of the islands across the sound from Seattle," I said, keeping the tone light and amazed at my own ability to speak her name in his presence after my weeks from hell.

"Oh, okay," he said, and let it drop.

Something had shifted. And a good thing too, for there was yet more on the horizon and life was about to take us to corners we had never entertained.

* * *

Just about the time I came together with Shari and found, at last, a quiet resolution about our friendship, another chapter in my life was simultaneously splintering. SFA, our spiritual community, began falling apart. After MSI's passing, the organization split into different groups, some interpreting his teachings one way and others another way. We, as householders, were caught in the middle, unsure where our loyalties should lie. We kept ascending, but began looking into other spiritual communities and other paths. It felt like an important transition point.

At this moment, it felt almost like we were back to the position we had been before the journey had commenced. Was that it? *Are we done? Have we gone as far as this journey can take us?* And even as I reflected I knew the answer was no. The journey thus far had given me a glimpse into living from a more authentic place, had shown me the thrill of staying open and vulnerable, but I was still filled with uncertainties as to my own worth, still attached to conditions I believed had to be met in order to be happy, and I still harbored plenty of fear. I wasn't sure what was next, but had experienced enough synchronicities at this point to trust that more would undoubtedly be revealed, if only I stayed alert and willing.

Personally, I hoped the "more" might involve some traveling. For the last several years, we had not gone on any adventures or traveled to any exotic locations, focusing our time and resources instead on attending ascension meditation retreats in the United States. Jake had been of the mind that we no longer needed to travel—that "hauling our carcasses around" would not get us any closer to enlightenment. But I missed our travels.

Then one day, seemingly out of the blue, Jake announced that he wanted to go to India. I absolutely jumped at the idea. Jake had been reading scores of Osho's books and decided he wanted to visit the Osho commune in Pune, India.

"Yes!" I cried. "Let's do it! It will be good to get away from the disorganization happening in the Ascension community. It will be an adventure!"

My little pixie self could hardly be contained.

Osho was a well-known, enlightened, albeit controversial mystic (aka Bhagwan Shree Rajneesh), who had been Margot Anand's teacher. Despite the controversy regarding his ashram in Oregon, we had read and greatly appreciated his syncretic teachings; the Osho Zen Tarot cards—which focus on gaining an understanding of the here and now, rather than the future, are based on the wisdom of Zen and the teachings of Osho, and point to the idea that events in the outer world reflect our own thoughts and feelings—had become important tools in my life. The Osho ashram in Pune, actually named the Osho International Meditation Resort, featured a "multiversity," and claims to be one of the largest centers in the world for meditation and personal growth processes. It offers classes or individual sessions in current Western therapy approaches, healing arts of East and West, esoteric sciences, creative arts, centering and martial arts, Tantra, Zen, Sufism, and meditative therapies. Programs range from one hour to three weeks.

A week later, we learned that a fellow ascender and travel agent was organizing a trip to India and could get us some discounts (more breadcrumbs?). Her group was going to be traveling to Sai Baba's ashram in southern India, and while we had no particular affinity with or interest in Sai Baba—an Indian spiritual master who was said to perform miracles—she urged us to check it out as well.

India! We decided that we needed to go for a month in order for the cost of the ticket and the travel time to be worth it. We also decided to invite Durga to go with us. Even though she had been a founding member of Ascension, she was less interested in the politics that emerged with its demise and more interested in continuing to explore the mystery of life—like us. Our friendship with her had blossomed over the past two years since our first Ascension retreats in North Carolina.

A couple of weeks into planning the trip, however, I suddenly panicked and decided it was just too much time away from the kids, who were only 8 and 11. We had been on numerous weekend retreats and had been away from the kids for 17 days, but a month? That was a long time.

We were sitting around the dinner table talking one night, a family ritual we did religiously from the time the kids were tiny all through high school, and I announced I didn't think I could go to India. It would be too hard to be away from them. There was a pause, and then Cassie said, very clearly and very sweetly, "Mommy, you *have* to go!"

Jacki looked at me and nodded in agreement. "You have to go."

I was confused. I had been expecting them to cheer when I announced my decision to stay home.

"Why do I have to go?" I asked.

Cassie said, "Because, Mommy, when Daddy first came up with the idea, you looked so happy and excited. We will be okay. Don't worry. It's only a month. The nanas and the grandpas always take really good care of us and we have fun. You have to go."

And with that, my daughters endorsed the trip, and we began planning in earnest.

The day before we were to leave for India, however, we were playing one of our favorite wrestling games with the kids, called "Get Daddy off the Mat!" We had a large gymnastics mat downstairs and the rules of our wrestling game were simple: we three girls had to get all of Jake's limbs off the mat. If we did so, we won, but if we didn't, he won. We'd been playing it for years and had never yet managed to get him off the mat, but there was always hope.

With our imminent departure, I think we girls ramped up the game a bit, determined to win this time. We got a little too rambunctious and one of the girls jumped onto Jake. He cried out and we abruptly stopped playing the game. We took Jake to the hospital and learned we had cracked one of his ribs . . . and we were leaving on an 18-hour plane trip taking us half way around the world the next day! Jake refused to give up on the trip, however, and refused to take any medication stronger than ibuprofen for the pain.

Later, Jake said it hurt with every breath he took. Then he told us it was the best thing ever, because it forced him to pay attention and be aware of every breath. If he stayed focused on his breath, his pain became a powerful meditation. He said he got high and happy traveling like that.

Chapter 22

Baba!

We have left on our journey to India amid tears of goodbye, last minute hospital visits, final soccer games and hurried packing. I feel curious as to this journey, nervous to leave the kids. It's always so bittersweet—the excitement of adventure, the pain of separation—like life itself. With each new challenge there is duality—the struggle of facing it and the silver linings within.
~ Journal entry, 28 October 2000

We rose the morning of our flight and boarded a Greyhound bus heading from Seattle up to Vancouver, British Columbia, where we would board our international flight to Amsterdam and then, after a 24-hour layover, head on to India. My mind was aswirl contemplating this next leg on our outer and inner journey. As we headed out on that cloudy morning, sitting on the dark-brown, speckled seats, gazing quietly out the window at the mottled gray Seattle sky, I began to contemplate what I hoped to gain from this trip. I still wanted to experience less fear, and I wanted to approach life with more innocence and trust—with the light-hearted, adventurous pixie spirit I had at 21. I also didn't want to waste any time on this precious journey—a whole month off from my responsibilities—how deep could I go? I wondered!

* * *

Never have I heard such a sound or seen such a sight. It was late afternoon and quite hot. We walked over to a coconut vendor to buy fresh coconuts and rest for a spell. A group of women were singing songs that drifted over the breeze. As we sat there we watched a thousand birds, probably mostly Indian myna birds, land on a large tree a little ways off. Mesmerized, we gazed as every branch became filled with birds, and then, as if in pure devotion to the moment and almost on cue, all the birds started singing, along with some women nearby. It was glorious, and it happened every afternoon at the ashram.

Sai Baba's compound, located in the tiny southern town of Puttaparthi, India, was a culture shock for us on many levels. We had no prior connection with or even knowledge about Sai Baba prior to heading down there with the small group of his devotees who had helped plan our trip. Pictures of him looked pretty strange with his large Indian Afro and bright-orange, floor-length robe. We learned that Sai Baba claimed to be the reincarnation of Sai Baba of Shirdi, a spiritual saint who died in 1918. At the time of our visit, he was famous for his reputed materializations of *vibhuti* (holy ash) and other objects, along with reports of miraculous healings. His devotees flocked to his ashram for *darshan*, a term which means "auspicious viewing," hoping to simply see Sai Baba, which in itself was considered a way to receive a blessing, but also hoping to witness one of his "miracles."

I had mixed feelings about these so-called miracles; it seemed to me that conjuring up ash could easily be a magician's trick. Miracles aside, however, Sai Baba had made an important contribution to India and elsewhere by urging his followers to undertake service activities as a means of spiritual advancement. Through his organization, an impressive network of free hospitals, clinics, drinking-water projects, and schools were established.

Dusty Puttaparthi itself was a strange mixture of Sai Baba

devotees, street vendors, and beggars. Especially memorable and delightful were the women who lined the streets with baskets piled high with gorgeous, fragrant, and colorful flower leis. They were everywhere and their presence perfumed the air with sweetness. At some point nearly every day, we would walk into town to purchase jasmine leis for the equivalent of 50 cents each. We would lavish these on ourselves, enamored with the powerful fragrance. As we walked through the streets that way, children and whole families would run after us, grabbing at Jake; invariably, he would take a whole gang of them to a fruit vendor and buy bananas for all.

Inside the walls of the ashram, a quiet prevailed, in marked contrast to the streets just outside the door. The grounds of the ashram were as impressive as its ornate and gaudy main temple, called Prasanthi Nilayam, "the abode of Highest Peace," which had the capacity to seat 15,000. There were numerous shrines and other temples within the ashram grounds, as well as a botanical garden, a bookstore, a library, and a spiritual museum. These last two contained the records of Sai Baba's life and works, and gave an overview of all the world's religions. There were also a sports complex and a planetarium, various accommodations, three canteens, a supermarket, a bakery, vegetable stalls, and an ice cream store.

We loved the beauty and the reverence of the place, but were not prepared for the segregation throughout the compound. Men and women did almost everything separately. In the canteens, there was a men's side and women's side; you were not allowed to eat together. At the supermarket, there were hours in which women could shop and different hours for men. At the temple, men and women were also physically separated; the men entered and were seated on one side, the women on the other.

We learned that Sai Baba preached a strict morality with regard to sensual desires, which encompassed food choices—no meat, no alcohol—and sex. He saw sexual interactions as a

stumbling block on the spiritual path and taught that any associ-
ation between sexes should be minimized. Jake and I were
allowed to sleep in the same room only because we were over 25
and had proof we were married. Otherwise we would not have
been permitted to sleep together. When we walked around the
compound we were not allowed to hold hands.

Durga had the hardest time of the three of us at the ashram.
Somehow, she was perceived as a threat to the women—a wanton
woman, perhaps? Durga is an extroverted, naturally gregarious
soul. She looks everybody in the eyes, and generally hails a
greeting when she sees someone she knows. At Sai Baba's, the
women were much more reserved. Eyes were downcast, and
body language was restrained. Women were expected to walk
behind men and to enter stores and temples after men. Durga
simply didn't fit in. When we would stand in line to go into the
temple for darshan, she would get admonished for some reason
or another, and often she was outright denied entry. There were
strict rules as to what you could wear and carry into the temple,
and she had a hard time following the rules to the letter.
Although bare bellies were acceptable, women were not
supposed to have any portion of their arms or legs exposed, and
the derriere was supposed to be covered by *two* layers of clothing.
Invariably, Durga's shawl would be too small or her shirt too
short. It was obvious, however, that she was singled out. On the
last day, she endeavored to do everything right. She made sure
that her arms and legs were covered completely and that her shirt
was very long, but she still got called out. We both had identical
passport purses that we carried everywhere, slung across one
arm and shoulder. I passed the checkpoint in front of her with no
complaints, but they refused to let her in, this time claiming that
her purse was too big! Poor Durga. It just wasn't her place.

Jake, however, was a phenomenal hit at the ashram, probably
because he wore all white and had long, thick, blond hair
streaming down his back, and always had flower leis on; he

looked like a *sadhu*—an ascetic, wandering monk. People would call out "Baba!" to him, which is a term of respect or endearment.

We spent the first day there touring the compound and learning all the rules. I was impressed by the fact that the compound was supported by all kinds of people offering various simple services for mere pennies: 20 people hovered around us clamoring to carry our seven bags for the equivalent of 50 cents, others offered bovine-pulled rickshaw rides, some sold fresh coconuts they opened for drinking. The scenes were like something from another century. While I found the grounds beautiful and stirring, I was also disturbed by the strange confluence of quiet reverence and rampant poverty, the jarring, outdated cultural traditions requiring segregation of the sexes, and an apparent agreement that women were somehow second to men.

We headed back to the dorm after dining separately, thankful that we would at least be allowed to sleep together. As we approached the dorm, I saw a woman and her young daughter seated on the ground before the entrance. They had spread a large blanket on the bare earth. They were poised in the midst of piles of carefully folded clothes, pulling more clothes from bags behind them and folding those, too. Puzzled by the scene, I stopped for a moment, trying to figure out what they were doing and why they were there. As I watched, the woman hailed another passerby, pointed to his clothes and made washing motions with her hands. I realized that she was offering a clothes-washing service. I was about to nudge Jake and suggest that maybe we should take her up on her service when she reached over to her young daughter, and with an unfolded piece of clothing in her lap, began picking at her daughter's head. It took me a minute to understand what was going on. She continued picking and pulling at strands, and wiping her hands in her lap, then taking up the activity again. Suddenly it dawned on me: *She's picking lice out of her daughter's hair!*

An inadvertent, tiny "Gross!" escaped my mouth as I pulled Jake in a wider circle far from her blanket. I quaked a little as I imagined how close I had just come to getting our clothes infested with lice.

What were we doing here? I had no feeling of connection to Sai Baba going in, only minor curiosity; we had come only because it was part of our travel agent's itinerary. Now that I was here I was filled with a sense of dismay over the segregation of sexes and shunning of any public display of affection, not to mention the prospect of lice. I couldn't help but wonder if there was really anything here for me.

We made our way safely into the dormitory, which was of a somewhat higher standard than the rest of the compound, since entry was only permitted to people who had paid to stay there. Having been reprimanded earlier for holding hands, we were happy to be beyond the judging eyes in the courtyard and relieved to be able to hug each other openly, as we were accustomed to doing.

Previous tenants had painted colorful murals on some of the walls. Our room had a beautiful rendition of Krishna playing his flute in front of a bovine bedecked remarkably like the ones in the compound, still pulling carts thousands of years later. I snapped a photo of Jake all decked out in a white *kurta pyjama* outfit (long white shirt and loosely gathered pants), a bright lei hanging around his neck, long hair streaming past his shoulders, the mural of Krishna playing the flute just behind him. Here, in a foreign land—in a religious ashram—surrounded by completely different cultural and spiritual traditions, it dawned on me that anything could happen. I fell asleep restlessly, half in resistance to being there, half curious what was next.

I startled awake. It was pitch black and I couldn't remember where I was. I felt afraid and started trembling, consumed with an overwhelming feeling that I had forgotten or missed something terribly important. As I lay there in the dark, craning my eyes to make out the edges of the room, I remembered that I was at Sai Baba's compound. My dream then came flooding back to me and I began laughing and crying in ecstatic gratitude. Sai Baba himself had appeared personally to me. It was as if he were actually there, talking to me. He had a message for me, which I had not understood during the dream, but now, the meaning flooded through me as I lay there and I understood: love really is letting go of fear. I recorded this event in my journal:

We've been at Sai Baba's ashram for 2 days now. The darshan has been rather inconsequential, however I did have a transforming experience here.

The first night I could hardly sleep but somewhere along the way I slipped into a dream. I dreamt that Maria led a small group of us to a door. She knocked and Baba said to come in. I remember thinking how easy that was . . .

Baba had his eyes closed but called out that the woman who was a teacher—yes the teacher woman—was to come sit by him. As Durga walked by he said he meant her. Then Baba said something that sounded like "the daughter of Durga" should come. We were all momentarily at a loss, then he smiled and said "oh you thought I said 'daughter of Durga' but I said 'dog of Durga'," referring to an incident earlier in the dream where Jake had pretended to be Durga's loyal dog—a private joke of sorts. We all laughed and Jake barked his way to Sai Baba's side. The dream Baba then turned to me and said "Mariah, you come up here too." I was all of a sudden at a loss that he knew my name, that he knew about the dog joke, and although I went up to him, inside I froze.

He turned to me, opened his eyes and said "tell me what you know is the way in" or something like that. I couldn't think. I tried to remember what I knew but just felt ill prepared for the question—like I was failing a test. I stammered something about you have to know your heart. He looked at me and said, "You can do better than that." I didn't know what to say or do. I wanted out of my skin. I started a stream of consciousness onslaught about "you have to live, love, play; you have to have fun," I said.

Then all of a sudden I was awake in our room at the ashram. Still trembling, with the fear of not knowing what I was supposed to know. I lay there feeling that way until from one moment to the next I suddenly knew what had been eluding me.

I started laughing and crying in ecstasy. I realized that all I had to do was not have fear—all I had to let go of was fear. It was so simple. Love is letting go of fear. So long ago I had read that and wondered about it and now here I knew it. I breathed it.

Now, as I write it, the impact of <u>that</u> moment is not here, but I know that I knew it and that thus, it is a part of me. (Journal entry, 3 November 2000)

A little later, I mentioned my dream to Maria who had arranged the trip. She looked at me, astonished.

"You dreamed that Sai Baba came to you?" she asked.

"Yes. It was quite amazing, actually. It was most definitely a spiritual dream." I started telling her about it.

"Well, yeah!" she said. "Didn't you know that a dream like that is something all Sai Baba devotees hope for?"

"What? To dream of him?" I asked, puzzled.

"Yes! You see, it is said that it is impossible to dream of Sai Baba unless he wills it."

"Really? But I had barely even heard of him," I argued. "And, no offense, but I don't really feel any connection."

She shrugged. "I don't know what to tell you. It's a rare and special thing to dream of him. You have been honored."

I had no idea what to make of this new information. While I couldn't deny that my dream had been tremendously important to me, I also couldn't fathom that he had willed himself into my dream state, and I couldn't reconcile his status as a guru against my feelings of unease over the segregation and possible inequality of the sexes there at the Sai Baba ashram.

A few days later, we went into the temple for evening darshan the last time, still hoping to see Sai Baba and possibly one of the famed "miracles" he was supposedly known for. One of the most honored and revered demonstrations by Sai Baba is that of producing vibhuti during darshan. Vibhuti is sacred ash used in Vedic rituals. Sai Baba taught that vibhuti is symbolic of detachment and renunciation, and that this means one's mind must become pure—desireless and detached—to be offered to God. During the evening darshan, occasionally Sai Baba would demonstrate this "miracle" for the crowd by selecting one recipient to stand up and offer their open palm, into which Sai Baba would make vibhuti appear.

At this darshan, there were about five to ten thousand people in attendance, and we were excited to see Sai Baba himself appear. We sat in our gender-designated sections and took in the ceremony, which, from my perspective, largely consisted of Sai Baba wandering about and talking a little.

From the women's side of the temple we could not see the men, but I learned afterwards that on that day Sai Baba had decided not only to appear, but also to demonstrate the vibhuti miracle to the men. Jake told us what happened when we got back together.

"I was sitting in the middle of the room near the front, while Sai Baba was walking around. After a little bit, he stopped by me and looked me in the eye. It was kind of confusing. I didn't really know what was going on and couldn't understand anything that anyone was saying, but the guy next to me nudged me, motioning me to lean forward and extend my hands out, cupped, palms facing up. So I did that. The next thing I knew, Sai Baba clapped his hands and rubbed them together over my hands, sprinkling them with something that looked like white ash. Some other guy started excitedly motioning that I should lick my palms. I did, but I guess I didn't get every last bit because the guy next to me grabbed my hands and licked them too."

We weren't sure whether or not the production of vibhuti was a miracle, but it did seem miraculous to us that not only were we in attendance on a day that he decided to do a demonstration, but that out of the thousands of men in attendance, other foreigners included, even a few white-skinned ones, Jake alone was selected to receive the blessing. What were the odds of that?

* * *

The three of us left Sai Baba's via hired car (think smelly old, little sedan with crazy driver—not chauffeur-driven limo). We were headed to Bangalore, four hours away. What a strange side trip that was. I had no idea what to make of the whole culturally jarring, yet spiritually significant experience. Maybe I never would. I watched the beautiful Indian countryside, and though I squealed with delight when we saw a bunch of monkeys, I also silently reflected that if ever there was an opportunity to overcome fear, as my Sai Baba dream had made clear, this little car ride was a good place to start. The drive was terrifying. I was used to people driving on their own side of the road. This driver, however, had no such conditioning and rarely bothered to stay on the correct side of the road; we barreled along as fast as his car could travel and had several near misses, by mere inches, with oncoming cars. His reckless driving was underscored when we saw a newly dead man on the side of the road, a few passersby hovering over him. How do you let go of perfectly reasonable fear?

After two hours, we stopped, frazzled, at a small town for a drink. We were the only foreigners. An old beggar woman with completely gray hair, dressed in a bright-orange silk sari and mustard-yellow belly shirt, approached us. In exchange for a few rupees she allowed me to take her photo. In the little café, the locals were fascinated and actually sat down at our table with us. We were as strange to them as they were to us. *How much of our impression of reality is solely due to cultural conditioning?* I wondered.

Chapter 23

Becoming a Sannyasin

I would like my sannyasins to live life in its totality, but with an absolute condition, categorical condition: and that condition is awareness, meditation.

~ Osho

The road trip, while long and somewhat harrowing, and the subsequent flight to Pune provided a much-needed transition from the Sai Baba ashram to the Osho ashram, for these were two very different animals. The Sai Baba crowd was strictly moral, reserved, and primarily Indian, and the Sai Baba grounds were quietly reverent amid normal activities. In contrast, the Osho ashram was composed of a highly cosmopolitan crowd, whose reverence came out in rambunctious, bubbling-over joy—a celebration of life, love, sex, and joy shared over lattes in the outdoor espresso café.

The Osho ashram lies in the middle of Pune, which is a sprawling metropolis—the ninth largest in India. We loved visiting the abundant street vendors who sold colorful clothing and semi-precious rocks on every corner. While Jake pored through bowls of lapis lazuli, moonstone, sunstone, labradorite, rose quartz, mother of ruby, and sugilite, I rifled through piles of silk saris and goddess clothing. Our suitcases were laden with these prizes when we went home. Today, I still put on goddess parties, where we dress up in these saris or gowns, and every room of our house bears witness to the rocks we collected on that trip.

We weren't allowed to stay overnight inside the ashram, so we found ourselves a hotel room, and later, a small apartment to stay in. Our little furnished apartment was decorated simply and served us well. It was tiny, maybe 30 feet by 30 feet, but there was a small bedroom, which cost extra for the bed, while Durga slept on a mat on the floor. It had a small living room/kitchen, a bathroom, and a tiny little balcony, where we would often find Durga in the morning, as it offered her a small space of her own.

Durga and I laughed until we cried about the toilets in Pune, most of which were two footprints over a hole next to a bucket for the paper, but some of which sprayed our nether regions with water and left us dripping.

Shortly after we had moved to our apartment on the quieter side of the ashram, we were walking back at the end of the day, still wearing our long maroon robes, which were required attire inside the ashram. I had been bemoaning the heat, how hard it was to breathe, and how I was getting a cold. I looked away from Jake and Durga momentarily and happened to catch a lone street vendor's eye. He was dressed all in white and had a stately presence. Cherubic brown cheeks peeked over a graying mustache; his eyes sparkled. "Coconut," he said, smiling and handing one to me. "Good for you!" I took the coconut, full of gratitude, and sucked hungrily at the straw. Oh, it was so refreshing, so healing. It was like I could feel that liquid hydrating my body and rallying my immune system. I knew it was good for me. (This was long before coconut water became a health fad in the US.) After that day, we would stop by the coconut stand every afternoon on the way home. The vendor would cheerfully lop off the top of the coconut, insert a straw, and with a little bobble of his head and a sweet, partially toothless smile, hand me a coconut. I loved that "coconut man."

Despite its colorful vendor charm, Pune is noisy, crowded, and terribly polluted by the inefficient, motorized rickshaws running this way and that everywhere. Every day, we walked back and forth to the commune in all that pollution.

Inside the Osho ashram is a lush tropical oasis set on a 28-acre campus with white marble pathways, elegant black buildings, abundant foliage, and an Olympic-sized swimming pool—a lovely sanctuary inside the polluted bustle of Pune. At its heart is an outdoor espresso café. My kind of place! We would gather there every morning, sipping our lattes among the voices of seekers from 20 different countries, all cheerfully chatting and laughing. At night we participated in the evening meditation meeting, which took place in a massive, marble-floored auditorium. Everyone wore white. The evening started with ten minutes of high-energy dancing, where we were invited to dance with pure abandon to beautiful, live spiritual music. The musicians would stop playing abruptly (and on purpose), at which point you dropped to the floor to sit quietly. After that, everyone sat in silence and watched an enormous video of Osho speaking. Initially, I thought the video part was kind of corny, but I came to appreciate it. His voice was mesmerizing, even via video; I often fell asleep.

Mostly, I loved those ten minutes of dancing. I would twirl like a whirling dervish across the massive floor and lose myself in some intrinsic form of spiritual dancing my body knew of its own accord, in which my fingers and arms would begin curving and twisting in front of me and above my head, and my body would undulate slowly. Everyone danced alone, not with partners, although sometimes I played with my white shawl as if it was a partner I was seducing. I closed my eyes and lost myself—feeling like poetry in motion—so alive. Jake beamed at me from time to time, and I at him, both appreciating the freedom of expression. More than one person came up to me afterwards and asked me where I learned to dance. I had no answer.

We participated in several different programs or sessions at the Osho ashram, but one that stood out for me was on shaman-istic healing. I did an individual session, and subsequently Jake and I took a beginning class. I had not received any energy healings before and was very curious about how the healer worked on you without ever touching your body.

At my first session, I entered the small room, which had a mattress that covered the entire floor space. The walls of the high-ceilinged room were light-colored and bare, except for small windows way up high that let a little natural light into the room and provided a view of blue sky and tiny fluffs of clouds. I lay on my back on the cushioned floor and the shaman quietly touched her hand to my chest. She never touched me again until the very end, when she put her hand back on my chest, to signify the session was over. I kept my eyes closed during the session, except for a brief peek, during which she was waving her hands in the space above and around me. During the session, and inextricably, my body began thrashing out of my control and actually lifted off the bed several times. I had no control over the movements of my body and no idea what to make of this, but as I personally experienced it, I could not deny that it happened, either. It was extraordinarily powerful. It was like someone had turned on the lights to an entirely different realm of existence. In my previous reality, it simply wasn't within the scope of possibility that one person could cause another person's body to move without physically touching them. It made me incredibly curious about shamanism and was a key factor in my later decision to study with a Toltec shaman. Also, since I knew this woman at Osho's was a student of Osho, it made me curious about him, too.

Over the course of the last few years I had become somewhat familiar with Osho through his books and the Osho Zen Tarot cards. I had grown to appreciate the readings and wisdom contained in the teaching book that came along with the cards and had gotten in the habit of drawing cards and doing readings for myself with some regularity to give me a focus for the day. Although I had stopped drawing Osho cards while we were at Sai Baba's, I decided to draw another card while we were here. It was a card that only appears in the Osho Zen Tarot deck—an extra Major Arcana card called "The Master," and it pictures Osho himself, which is now sketched into my journal. The card read:

> You are caterpillars—**bodhisattvas**. All caterpillars are bodhisattvas and all bodhisattvas are caterpillars. A bodhisattva means one who can become a butterfly, who can become a buddha, who is buddha in the seed, in essence . . . (Major Arcana, "The Master" card, Osho Zen Tarot (1994), p. 47)

As I read the description below the picture, I remembered the first day of love and ecstasy training when I watched a caterpillar crawl the length of the meeting room, and again I sensed the potential for transformation.

* * *

On the last day before we left the Osho ashram, I made a spontaneous decision to participate in the initiation ceremony to become a sannyasin, which Osho describes as a decision "to live life in its totality, but with an absolute condition, categorical condition: and that condition is awareness, meditation."

I was drawn to his words: "I teach my sannyasins to celebrate everything . . . I celebrate life. It brings unhappiness – good. I celebrate it. It brings happiness – good, I celebrate it. Celebration is my attitude, unconditional to what life brings."

I loved that Osho embraced all of life and that I could choose to also. I knew that participating in this ceremony was a commitment to myself to deliberately, consciously search for truth and for God by diving headfirst into life with passion, intensity, awareness, and acceptance.

In the small room where the ceremony was held, I waited with the others who had decided to go through the ceremony.

Neither Jake nor Durga chose to participate, but they were there supporting me, waiting for me. Durga helped me dress up for the occasion. I donned a red and black, floor-length goddess gown covered in black sparkles. I had bought it at a boutique in Bombay, unaware at the time that I would have this occasion to wear it, and as a final touch Durga put an Indian *bindi* in the middle of my forehead—a classic Indian decoration that represents the third eye, or seat of concealed wisdom.

In the throng, I felt nervous, although the ceremony was exceedingly simple. You simply waited your turn in line and approached the leaders one at a time. The sannyasin group leaders held your gaze and, from what I could tell by watching others, they might or might not say something to you. They handed you a piece of paper, which would bear a spiritual name—a sort of guidance for what was important for your growth, as I understood it.

I barely remember the ceremony. I can't recall if I said or repeated words or vows, but I remember that when I walked up to the woman leading the ceremony to receive my scroll with my new name, I looked deeply into her eyes. Since soul gazing was a big part of my practice, she surprised me when she said to me, "Close your eyes—your focus is too outward—go inside." I closed my eyes and could feel the subtle shift inward. This was where I needed to go.

Durga and Jake were grinning ear to ear and placed an abundance of jasmine leis around my neck to honor this rite of passage.

"So, what is your sannyasin name?" Jake asked excitedly.

I looked at him shyly, and unrolled the scroll. "It says, 'Ma Bodhi,'" I said.

Durga looked at me and grinned. "Ahhh," she said, "that means 'awakening.' Sounds like it is time for the next step."

I sat there glowing like a newlywed, but inside I was nervous. Was I really ready for the next step?

Chapter 24

Writing My Way Home

I must always choose my passion, whatever the danger. And my passion invariably involves reams of paper.
~ Elizabeth J. Andrew

Passion.

I thought about the word a lot when we got back from India. And I could barely think of it without thinking of writing. Some people sing, some dance or do sports and, while I dabbled in all those things, what I had always been most passionate about was writing. True, I had shied away from writing for publication—from writing for others—for many years, unsure I had anything worthy to say, but I never stopped writing for myself.

There was something about writing that moved me. And freshly back from taking sannyas—from dedicating myself to living passionately with awareness and acceptance—I turned my attention to examining my passion for writing. What was it about writing that moved me so?

In my journals at this time, I wrote:

Anne Lamont says in "Bird by Bird" that sometimes you do a tea ceremony because you want the caffeine and then it turns out it was the tea ceremony after all that you wanted. I think writing is like that for me. Do I want to write some wonderful piece that inspires the whole world—or is it just the ceremony of the writing that I want to get back to?

> I don't like so much to make up stories. I like to write what I see here and now—sometimes it helps me see.
> (Journal entry, September 2001)

I began to notice that the act of writing seemed to bring me closer to the moment. When I wrote I slowed down and paid more attention. And when I wrote about myself in my journals, it gave me some distance from myself. I could witness my feelings more easily. I could let loose without pre-editing everything. I wrote in my journal:

> Writing is a lot like ascension. All we want to do is get back to the business of getting out of the way. Some days that seems simply impossible. There've been days, I won't say how many, where I've called one of the teachers and told them this time I am really stuck.
>
> They'll pause quietly and say "Are you ascending? Are you choosing?" but I'll just wail "I'm just so depressed!"
>
> "So?" I'll hear back. "What's wrong with being depressed?"
>
> I hate that when they say that—it inevitably makes me feel better and really I was so thoroughly enjoying being depressed . . . except, of course, for the depressing part.
>
> So, why do I want to write? Because for a few moments I get out of my own way.

Hunched over another one of my multitudinous journals, I contemplated what I might write about, if I wrote for others. I had always been drawn to writing non-fiction rather than fiction. *But what expertise do I bring to the table?* I asked myself. *What do I really "know"?* I rolled this thought over in my journal:

> Write what you know, experts always say. Trouble is, as I go through life, I know less and less; very disconcerting that is, I must say.

I know a lot about crying and quite a bit about sex.

I know doubt. I know fear. I know jealousy. I know insecurity and lack of self worth. I know self-judgment and judging others.

I know what it feels like to be rejected and abandoned.

I know what it feels like to be present.

Hmm . . . again what I know best is crying and orgasm . . . Oh and I'm really scared half the time.

(Journal entry, September 2001)

And it was true. At this time, even though I had experienced so much healing, even though I had forgiven and was full of gratitude, I still felt fear and shame. And I cried. A lot. My inner critic felt like by this time in the journey, six years after the events that launched me, after enormous heart-opening events and prophetic dreams, I should be a picture of serenity and peace projecting a calm exterior that reflected pools of silence within. More to the point, I should know *something* more than crying and orgasm. But both inwardly and outwardly, on any given day, I was a hot mess. Who wants to read about that?

Looking for answers, I kept drawing and reading Osho Zen Tarot cards too. My journals are sprinkled with drawings of different cards. Right in the middle of this journal that was all about writing and crying, I had drawn a picture of the card I had picked during a reading. The card was called "Ice-olation." The picture is of a man encased in ice. Only his face is showing with rainbow-colored tears streaming down his face. The card's commentary says this:

The rainbow-colored tears on this person's face hold the key to breaking out of this "ice-olation". The tears, and only the tears, have the power to melt the ice. It's okay to cry, and there is no reason to feel ashamed of your tears. Crying helps us to let go of pain, allows us to be gentle with ourselves, and finally helps us to heal.

The disconnect became clear. On some deep level I was ashamed that I still cried so much. Never mind that my tears often formed from gratitude rather than pain, never mind that I experienced release myself when I cried. The bottom-line message from my secret hateful self was: I cried too much. The unconscious follow-through was therefore I am still broken; therefore I have nothing to offer others.

But at this juncture, I did have something new to offer *myself*: my commitment to living passionately with awareness and acceptance. Writing, I came to see, was an integral part of that commitment. First I was passionate about writing. Second, writing, like meditation, increased my capacity for awareness. Writing took me out of my scorpion-focused self, giving me the chance to closely examine my life, shining the light on unconscious thoughts still programming me.

And acceptance? Well, a commitment to acceptance required that I accept whatever the path looked like, hot mess or not. I did not know where the path was leading, or if there was a resolution, but in following my passion to keep writing, I gave myself permission to experience it—to keep exposing the unexposed. I wrote:

> I've been fed up with myself, fed up with others. I've cried buckets both in real life and on paper. Yet, still, even still with nothing to say, with no story to tell, I write.
> (Journal entry, September 2001)

Something may have been bursting to come out, but it was the process that was most important, or, as Elizabeth J. Andrew says in *Writing the Sacred Journey*, "Writing is the means, not the end . . . You can only discover why a story matters by telling it or writing it."

Ultimately, in order to share any of it, I would have to follow my passion, find myself worthy, and write my way home.

Chapter 25

Shamanic Initiation

It's not that we fear the place of darkness, but that we don't think we are worth the effort to find the place of light.
~ Hugh Prather

Although the Ascension community at large was still struggling and fighting, we discovered that our little core group of householders was content to continue meeting and ascending together once a week at each other's houses. We all wanted and needed more support, however, and began to read other spiritual books available at the time, even while continuing to ascend regularly.

We were very fortunate to live in the Seattle area at the time, because many great teachers passed through, and we had the good fortune to hear a number of phenomenal, enlightened people speak, each of whom touched us. We loved hearing Byron Katie, author of *Loving What Is*. And while we did not participate in her longer workshops, we did practice her work, which gently encouraged us to examine our thoughts, especially our thoughts of judgment, to see how they might be conditioning and affecting our life, and also to see if they might not actually be reflections of that which we feared or hated most about ourselves.

We also saw and sat with Eckhart Tolle, who wrote *The Power of Now*. Sitting in that room with Eckhart was a powerful experience. He said very little, yet filled the room with a great presence. The air got thick and syrupy, and my own thinking slowed until I, too, was quiet inside. Eckhart's book is one of those we always keep near and read from regularly.

Another impressive man we met was Don Miguel Ruiz, who wrote *The Four Agreements: A Practical Guide to Personal Freedom*. Ruiz reminded us to "be impeccable with your word, don't take anything personally, don't make assumptions, always do your best." His book was advertised as a book of Toltec wisdom, and this intrigued us greatly because of Jake's experience reading the Carlos Castaneda books. We were not particularly drawn to study more directly with Ruiz, but we did become interested in learning more about Toltec shamanism, especially since I had had such a powerful experience in India. We began to appreciate the larger picture and to see that there were other paths all pointing in the same direction, each with a slightly different emphasis.

Right around this time, Merilyn Tunneshende's book came out, *Don Juan and the Art of Sexual Energy: The Rainbow Serpent of the Toltecs*. Here was a title that totally jumped out at us: serpents, sexual energy, and Carlos Castaneda's teacher? Who was this woman? We learned quickly that she was a Toltec sorceress and "Nagual." (Nagual is a term used by Carlos Castaneda to refer to a person who has the skills to guide people to new areas of awareness and alternate realities.) We learned that Tunneshende had been taught "dream power" (energetic healing and sorcery) over the course of a 20-year apprenticeship in the Mexican desert with the same Nagual sorcerers, including Don Juan, who had taught Carlos Castaneda. And, we learned, she was going to be leading a four-day workshop on Vashon Island in Seattle on shamanic dreaming. We immediately signed up. The workshop was to be held at the Trillium Retreat Center on Vashon Island.

Vashon Island was a 15-minute ferry ride from Seattle— just the right distance to feel like you'd gotten away from it all without spending hours traveling. The Trillium Retreat Center was situated on 15 acres of land that was a combination of forests and meadows, with little trails through the woods to different outbuildings, including a yurt at the end of one trail through the woods, a bathhouse, complete with an outdoor hot tub, a Russian steam bath, and a cold plunge down another path. There was a communal dining hall where we ate, and a large yurt where we met. The accommodations were rustic cabins set in a small clearing in the woods, each with four sets of bunks; men and women slept separately, even Jake and I.

Merilyn's workshop was not like any other I had been to. While she lectured and taught us about different concepts and helped us to identify our intentions, as one might expect, each day she would also assign us homework (bunkwork, I guess), which itself was not unusual. But this homework was to be accomplished in the middle of the night. In fact, every couple of hours, someone wielding a rattle would awaken us to encourage us to drift in and out of a dream state more often during the night. We were to practice remembering our dreams, to write them down, and to pay attention to the symbolism that came through our dreams, especially right at the moment we were waking up. There were other tasks to do as well. She would give us instructions that required us to leave our bunks in the middle of the night and travel somewhere in the woods, generally to the yurt, to complete an activity. If someone was already present in the yurt when we got there, we were to quietly step to the side and wait outside until they were finished.

We hoped to have "lucid" dreams. I have had this experience a number of times in my life and it is unforgettable and unmistakable. In lucid dreaming you become aware—that is fully conscious—while dreaming. Usually the experience involves something your waking brain knows is impossible, such as you are flying, or you are talking with your dead father. The intensity of lucidity can vary greatly, from not only being aware that you are dreaming, but also to knowing that there is no real danger; you can learn to alter your dream while it's happening, too. Merilyn taught that there was yet another realm to dreaming, called dream bridging, where you use your dreams to help manifest things or ideas or even people.

The first night our dreaming task was to discover our root attachment or agreement—some unconscious agreement we had made with ourselves that might have been keeping us from growing. In order to do this we were to think about it as we fell asleep and then at some point during the night, we were to leave our bunks and make our way to the yurt where she had placed a red and black bowl with a piece of obsidian in it. We were to peer into the obsidian in search of our root attachment or agreement. Later, we were to submerge ourselves in the lunar pool (an outdoor Jacuzzi) to discover it. I kept notes about my experience during this retreat and wrote:

> At the lunar pool, while Merilyn was speaking, I felt a flash of "attachment to death," rather than to life—it was unexpected.
> As I begin my journey to falling asleep, I am thinking, wondering what my root agreement is. I see myself swimming past "loss of innocence," being surrounded by taking care of others, strength . . . attached to people who are asleep, to the sleeping world, to making sure they are okay . . . to being understood . . . to mediating.
> (Journal entry, 30 August 2002)

After the first rattle, I made my way to the yurt in the pitch black of night and peered into the bowl, but it took great effort and nothing happened. I wrote that I was "holding on, not seeing clearly." I went back to my bunk and just before I fell asleep I thought I heard someone singing or moaning in the woods. Then I fell asleep and dreamed I went to the lunar pool. My dream held interesting symbolism:

> I dreamed that this group was having a party of sorts, maybe an after workshop celebration. I volunteered to put "Heart"

[the name of a young boy in my dream] to bed. I did so then went to go to the lunar pool. Just as I was about to get in, I realized he was back up and was wandering near the swimming pool. I was torn by my desire to go in the tub and being worried and feeling responsible about him.

It was not a lucid dream, but just as I was waking up, I almost became lucid in the dream. I remember someone handing me a purple swirly psychedelic cover for a slug bug car.

(Journal entry, 30 August 2002)

When I woke up, I initially couldn't remember anything about my dream except for a purple psychedelic slug bug, but when I headed out for real to the lunar pool, it came back to me and I wrote it down. I returned to my bunk. Just before the second rattle I dreamed that Merilyn came to me and asked me sharply if I got the message from the ancient Chinese. Her question tickled something, but I couldn't pull it up and was very sleepy. She said, "We're wasting our time if you don't get it." I woke later and realized that I was somehow committed to staying asleep. The rattlers came around a third time and I woke up thinking about Merilyn's dream message. I wrote: "I don't know what the message is but I keep thinking about a thousand-year-old egg and I saw Buddha."

I decided to return to the yurt to gaze once again in the bowl. I saw then that one of my root agreements was not to wake up fully. I now perceived that this was because I felt I was needed in the regular world to take care of others, to take responsibility, but I also saw that there was pride involved. I was holding on to an agreement of martyrdom. Essentially, I was choosing not to be fully alive, in the name of some sort of glorified self-sacrifice. Suddenly, I was clear that this was because I had misunderstood how I was needed.

The course of the night's activities had revealed 1) an

attachment to death, rather than life; 2) an attachment to not seeing clearly; 3) an attachment to making sure everyone else was okay and to not waking up, because I was needed; and 4) an attachment to self-sacrifice and martyrdom.

When I summed these up I could see that my unconscious root agreements had left me unclear about how to serve and how to live, and that as a result, I had unwittingly agreed to live a slow death in order to "take care" of others.

It occurred to me that the world needs people to take risks and to be fully alive, embracing life, not shying from it—selfless, perhaps—but not mired in martyrdom. We had been taught that particularly potent dream messages typically came in the gap between waking and sleeping—either right after falling asleep or at the moment when you were waking up. On the morning after my first night, just as I was waking from a dream, I heard the words "Come up you and find you," and wrote in my journal: "I choose the boat crossing the darkness."

* * *

Ask a direction for help in knowing how to proceed. Go to the yurt and supplicate to a direction.
~ Journal entry, 31 August 2002 (Day Two Instructions at Tunneshende Workshop)

Merilyn's instructions were always just beyond the grasp of my logical mind. Ask a direction for help? What does that mean? Supplicate to a direction? Huh? Still, I trusted her on some level and simply followed along as best as I could. We were to go to sleep and would be awakened by rattling. At some point in the night we were to get up and go to the yurt, asking a direction for help in how to proceed and then supplicating to that direction.

That night I didn't remember any dreams, but I remember thinking just before I fell asleep that it would be appropriate to give an offering to the "west" before supplicating it. Merilyn had taught us the importance of making offerings whenever you did a ritual and also offering ourselves to the group in the form of sharing our experiences.

Every day, after a night of following her instructions, we would gather in the yurt as a big group and go around the circle sharing our dreams, telling what had happened to us, and what we might have gleaned from any of the assignments. Jake and I were comfortable with group sharing both from love and ecstasy training and from our meditation retreat. Even so, sharing the next day after that particular instruction was given was one of the more difficult things I have ever done.

I'd had a potent experience that seemed wildly out of context for this particular group. Still, I knew I had to share with as much authenticity as I could muster. On the last day everyone has an opportunity to share with the group as the final joint activity. I decided to read from my journal, where I had recorded the night's activities immediately afterwards, still reeling from the experience myself. Sitting on my knees with my head bowed, I began reading from my journal, shaking with the memory of the event, but also shaking with trepidation at saying out loud to this group what I had written:

I headed to the yurt where someone was already worshipping. I stepped to the side behind the bench and rested in child's pose. I meditated and remembered I hadn't brought any offerings. I knew I couldn't enter without them. I returned to the hut and gathered up the antlers, the love candle, 2 crystal wands and a sunstone. I found a blue lace agate already in my bag . . .

I asked for guidance.

My supplication took on a life of its own. I inserted the laser [quartz crystal] wand and entertained the possibility of orgasm. As I went deeper to the source and asked for help, I heard these words: "Don't look back." I lost all shame and cranked up my own heat. I gave it my all, feeling as if I were being made love to by a consuming fire

—FUCKED BY FIRE—

I begged for new birth. I wanted that orgasm to result in a new birth.

The laser wand I had inserted was hot when I removed it. (Journal entry, 31 August 2002)

Tears were streaming down my face and the room was stunned to silence when I finished. Even Merilyn had no words and her expression was inscrutable, but Jake smiled kindly at me. Then, tentatively, a man raised his hand. He said, "I wasn't going to say anything because it had been so personal, but since she has spoken, I will say that I was there, and inadvertently witnessed her experience. I had just left my bunk to go to the yurt myself when I noticed someone was there. I moved to the side, to the bushes, but couldn't help but hear her as she was overcome by something more powerful than herself. It was moving to witness." I had no idea what to make of my experience or the sharing of it. The meaning was to come later.

By the end of the workshop, I had set a new intention: I wanted to go on the women's journey that Merilyn mentioned she was leading. We had learned over the last two days that Merilyn had two major journeys scheduled in the next two years. The first, scheduled for the coming December, was a women's journey where women from around the world would have an opportunity to participate in an ancient Mayan ceremony at the sacred sites (primarily Chichen Itza and Uxmal) of the Yucatan. It was a ceremony that had not been performed on-site for over 500 years, following first the Spanish conquistadors' conquest of the Yucatan and later Mexican independence. In both cases the indigenous Mayans were subjugated and their culture all but extinguished. The following year she would lead a men's journey.

The problem for me was that all the other women who were going had long been her students and had been preparing logistically and psychologically for some time. Still, I asked Merilyn if I could join the group, for I felt a strong calling. She said she would consider adding me to the group, but the deadline for all the money and travel arrangements was 4 September—only three days later. I would have to figure out how to overcome that hurdle on my own. That meant I would have to contact the coordinator, who lived in London, make all my own travel arrangements, get travel insurance, and pay in full immediately. I gasped. That seemed impossible. Merilyn was unperturbed and just said that if I really intended to be there, I would figure out how to make it happen.

Jake was 100 percent supportive and encouraged me to do whatever it took to go. As it turned out, the London coordinator was able to grant me a two-week extension to get my money and travel documents in order. Before the end of September, I had purchased plane tickets and travel insurance, had paid in full, and was confirmed for the journey.

What I didn't know at the time was that our life was about to turn upside down, again.

"Are you sitting down?" Jake said in a whisper one morning in October when he called me from work. There had been grumblings for some time following the acquisition of the small start-up he had been working for by a larger company. We knew something big was going down when he left for work that morning. We weren't sure if he would have a job by the end of the day.

"Oh no, did you lose your job . . .?" I faltered, thinking about our huge mortgage and my much lower-paying job.

"Uh, no—not exactly," he mumbled.

"Well, that's good. Right?" I pressed.

"Not sure," he said bluntly. "They fired about two-thirds of the workforce. I am one of the few that get to keep my job."

"But that's great!" I said enthusiastically, confused as to why he didn't sound happier.

He paused. "The job has been moved to North Carolina," he replied finally.

My heart skipped a beat.

"North Carolina? What? Why?"

Thoughts ran rampant through my head in those few moments. *But our family is all here in the Pacific Northwest.* My mind panicked as I tried to imagine moving. *Wait, we just bought this beautiful home less than two years ago. Now we're going to have to move again . . . and sell it? It's not a seller's market! North Carolina? After all those years of possibly moving to North Carolina to do teacher training with SFA, now work is moving us there, just as SFA is closing down? This is absurd!*

Jake broke through my haphazard thoughts. "They are going to fly us to North Carolina in two weeks to take a look. We have to make our decision by the end of the month. If we agree to go, they will fly the whole family out for a second visit in December to spend more time looking for a house." He paused, and then added, "For those of us remaining, they have sweetened the pot considerably. If we go, they have guaranteed us a premium over the appraised value of our house to ensure we don't lose money selling it in this market. Plus, they will pay all our moving expenses and pay for temporary housing in North Carolina while we look for a new house. Also, they have offered me a raise, and if I stay employed with them for another year, my stock will have vested."

"But we can't go . . . " I trailed off.

"I know. Everybody we love is here and I want to stay. But we are going to have to seriously think about it because there may not be any other jobs in my field available here . . . it's a terrible time. And, if we don't take their deal and they don't help us sell our house, we will be completely responsible for this huge mortgage—on your paycheck alone."

We tried for two weeks to come up with some option whereby we could stay, but in the end we couldn't do it; we couldn't say no to the generous offer we had been given to move, especially when balanced against the destitute financial situation if we stayed. We began to make arrangements to move across the country, including going out for the initial all-expenses-paid trip to North Carolina to see the lay of the land, the company's new digs, and to hear the pitch about why the Research Triangle Park in the Raleigh-Durham-Chapel Hill quadrant of North Carolina was a hotbed of innovation and opportunity.

On the last day of that trip as we were heading to the Raleigh airport to fly home, we went back to drive by a couple of houses we had seen. We stopped on the side of the country road to regroup for a minute. It was pouring—hot pelting raindrops—a novelty for us Seattleites. The air smelled like the tropical section of Seattle's Woodland Park Zoo, rich, humid and fertile. We had paused next to a driveway that was framed by a beautiful wisteria archway. Peeking through the archway, it looked like the gateway to a magical, enchanted forest. We couldn't quite see the house, only the driveway and then a winding boardwalk trail that curved out of sight through lush foliage. While I admired the charming setting, I spotted a wooden stake practically buried in the bushes. A sheet protector was nailed to it and there was a single white piece of paper inside. I jumped out of the car and grabbed it. It was a simple flyer with no photos, only a diagram of the property and the following words:

BY OWNER ON TIMBERLY DRIVE
Perfect for Nature or Animal Lovers

5.8 acres wooded and open with stable, aviaries, and other outbuildings

Rancher with finished basement

4 bedrooms, 2 bathrooms, 3000 plus square feet
Large Decks
Enclosed Porch
Hot Tub

Call 442-6656

"Look! This place is for sale!" I read the flyer out loud. "Oh, doesn't it look cool," I bubbled.

Jake got a funny, faraway look on his face. "Maybe I'll buy a ranch for our girls . . . " he said dreamily.

Then he abruptly came to. "Hey, we gotta go! We're going to be late to the airport. Keep that flyer. We can call the owner and talk to her when we get back home. We have a couple of months before you leave on the women's journey."

Chapter 26

Rainbow Women's Journey

Why am I here?
~ Merilyn's question for the Rainbow Women

I sat people-watching in the Seattle-Tacoma airport while waiting for my flight to Cancun, where I would meet up with the rest of the women participating in Merilyn's women's journey. I ended up talking with a woman who was going to be flying to Raleigh, North Carolina, on a connecting flight. At the mention of North Carolina, all the intensity of the past few months returned to me. We had made our decision. We were moving to Raleigh in three weeks!

The dates of my women's journey overlapped exactly with the dates of the second all-expenses-paid trip to North Carolina to go house shopping. Jake and the kids were heading there. They would have to pick out our new house without me. I thought about the pretty framed driveway we had seen on the last day. We had called the lady with the house for sale on the flyer and had begun a conversation, but of course we had not seen the house yet. She had sent us some photos and it was clear the house was a 45-year-old eclectic, tacky disaster: old scarred wood paneling, still older floor-to-ceiling metal shelving, an indoor/outdoor rug made to look like bricks in the living room, unpainted cement blocks downstairs, and a bathroom so tiny if you sat on the toilet your knees practically hit the back wall—not to mention, even, the built-in gigantic wooden waterbed contraption covered in faded red shag surrounded by linoleum made to look like rocks that had been cut in a wavy line as if to simulate a river bed stapled over hardwoods in the master bedroom.

Still, there was something about it that called to me. For one thing, the setting in the forest was bewitching, and the house was built to enjoy it, with large picture windows in the main rooms and a master bedroom with lots of windows to take in the forest on all sides, plus a big wood deck circling the house. On the west side a second, higher deck had been built to support a giant hot tub, so that you could soak in the forest as if in a tree house. Ivy threatened to engulf the backside of the house, giving it a magic cottage look. I wondered what the kids would think.

I brought my attention back to the women's journey, mulling over all the preparation I had made. In the three months preceding the journey, Merilyn had sent numerous instructions to the participants to help us ready ourselves. We had reading assignments that included her book and others, dreaming practices, and "recapitulation" practices. Recapitulation is a formal ceremony where you regather energy lost in the course of life. Sometimes you might lose energy by being hurt, but it can also happen simply through conditioning, where we live a certain way because it is what we are used to.

As I ramped up for the journey, I followed her instructions. I wrote about the process:

I am working my way the second/third time through the Art of Sexual Energy, having last read it completely a year ago and then partially before the Vashon Island Workshop. I have also been playing with recapitulation and today am working on formal recapitulation of the burdened and dethroned sacred feminine. It is an interesting journey. I am excited to continue this healing work. Two days ago, I had a strong dream about the upcoming journey. In the dream I was attending a special pre-journey gathering of attendees . . . Merilyn/Dona

212

Celestina wanted to tell me that I could not go on the journey because I was not ready because I had not detached from my husband and children. In that moment, I became very present in the dream and rather than reacting in fear of my failure, I told her honestly that I was not completely detached but that I was proceeding (evolving) toward that. I was very present. In the next moment she laughed and hugged me and let me know I could go.

(Journal entry, fall 2002)

I reflected on the importance of this dream. I knew this journey Jake and I were on was showing me the difference between commitment and attachment, between love and attachment. It had been an important theme for me during my Ascension retreats, and here it was coming up again. What was wrong with attachment? Didn't being attached to someone mean you were deeply bonded to them? That you were committed? That you loved them? I knew that was what I wanted. I wanted the deepest bonding possible with my beloved Jake. I wanted mystical union.

I read once that attachment ties us to the mundane and earthly, while love attaches us to the mystical and divine. I began to see that. Attachment has a "needy" aspect to it. It is about filling a void, meeting a need, and using someone else to feel better about ourselves. It is motivated by the fear of losing, rather than by love for the other person. My attachment to Jake made me want to control things to predict the outcome. I felt like I knew what was best for us and how to get there. But as I began to investigate the subtleties of love, commitment, and attachment, I began to see that it was my attachment—not my love, not my commitment—that often got in the way. My attachment was tied to a belief that I needed to be hyper-vigilant to keep Jake and me on track. It was reminiscent of my prior experience on planes, which was about me keeping all the passengers safe, a vigilance that gave way to freedom and enjoyment when I relinquished control to the pilot. I was beginning to see that I was going to have to let go of my attachment to Jake, and to consider that maybe I didn't know everything . . . maybe my way wasn't the best way . . . maybe I wasn't the pilot of our journey. Maybe it was time to trust: trust life, trust Jake, and trust something greater than myself.

Merilyn called us the "Rainbow Women." The rules of the journey were simple: be punctual, respect each other, and offer without expectation. We Rainbow Women were to spend some time throughout the course of our journey asking ourselves again and again, "Why am I here?"

On the first night, I returned to my room to ponder the question and wrote:

Why am I here?

Thinking back on the decision—the yearning to come—I recall the last workshop. In that fire orgasm I felt something. I felt myself. Also, in letting Jake completely stand on his own and watching him blossom, I felt a deep happiness and strength. I was proud of myself. I wanted more of that. I wanted more opportunity to stand on my own and to let others stand on theirs. Also the result was a feeling of deep connection and gratitude—a coming together from wholeness. That's what I want. I want to burn away that which doesn't serve. I want to be courageous and selfless and to allow the mystery to unfold. I want to be more aware of my energy body that I know exists. I want to contribute what I have to contribute. I want to feel at ease and strong. I want to let go of the little me. I want to let go of jealousy. I want to trust.

(Journal entry, 3 December 2002)

The next morning we set out on our journey by bus. We were

headed first for Uxmal, one of the most famous sacred sites of the Yucatan. After a couple days, we would continue on to Chichen Itza—the best-known sacred site of the region—with visits to ceremonial caves, Loltun and the Cave of the Jaguar Serpent, Balamkanche, on the way.

Along with Merilyn, who had been involved in Toltec-Mayan shamanism for 23 years, we would also be accompanied by Ana Maria, a teacher and ceremonialist who focused on the sacred feminine, and her husband, a former caretaker of Chichen Itza and student of Mayan shamans and Mayan cosmology. Most importantly, we would also be accompanied by a Mayan priestess from Belize named Maria Garcia, who was descended from the original Mayan priestesses who cared for the sacred sites in ancient times. She was also the niece of a beloved Mayan healer priest, Don Eligio Panti of Belize. Maria was coming along to perform a *primicia*, an ancient Mayan ceremony that was a ritualized expression of gratitude. Through these ceremonies the Mayans sought a relationship with the gods of the cosmos and the underworld, whom they believed controlled all the elements of life.

Merilyn told us it was highly unusual for a Mayan priestess to agree to come so far to be with a group of foreign women and that we were very fortunate. The ceremony Maria was recreating had not been allowed to be performed on-site at the Mayan sacred sites in hundreds of years due to politics, but Merilyn had been granted permission to take our group to particular areas of the sacred sites not usually open or accessible. The ceremony would take place over several days and included offerings of food and other things that each of us would contribute, most importantly an attitude of reverence and appreciation.

I couldn't help but think that while Maria would be working hard to remember and preserve her cultural heritage, I was here trying to forget mine, trying to look deeper. I wanted to be removed from the strings of my culture, my family, my roles so I could find my true core. Travel had always helped me to open up and soften.

One day on the bus, Merilyn was talking and we were asking questions. She was in the front of the bus when I asked my question. She didn't know me by name and I wasn't sure if she even recognized me, as I had only spent a couple of days with her previously. I don't remember what I asked, but she turned around and peered down the bus at me, then said, "Ah, it is the Tantrika asking." When she said that, I felt seen and accepted; I appreciated my unconventional path. Tantrikas are known for embracing all of life—for diving in and fully experiencing life, rather than repressing or rejecting any part of it. A Tantrika, it is said, uses the wisdom of her body and senses as a means to becoming more present, and works to bring compassion and light to every aspect of life. A Tantrika says "yes" to life in all its beauty and chaos: light and shadow, hard and soft, movement and stillness, masculine and feminine, lunar and solar. Here I was on a Toltec shamanism journey, but I was still on a Tantric path too.

Our first destination, Uxmal, was very fitting. In ancient times, Uxmal was a school of mysteries and spiritual ceremonies. It served as the largest university of spiritual wisdom for the whole of the Mayan empire. There was a particular structure called "The Nunnery." Miguel told us that scholars hypothesized that Mayan women engaged there in the study of various energy sources: feminine, sexual, lunar, and Kundalini energy. I felt connected in some kind of timeless, ageless, cultureless way.

Merilyn talked a lot about understanding and feeling the importance of this Mayan ceremony, and for feeling deep within ourselves as to why we were there. As she talked, I felt a sense of spinning a great web—of weaving a new tale to replace the old. Even though it was strictly a Mayan ceremony we were recreating, I felt that we were weaving a web of many diverse cultures. Interestingly, the word "Tantra" means weaving and expansion. Tantra reminds us that all the diverse threads of our experience are part of the whole and holy tapestry of life. It's easy to embrace beauty and joy, but it's much harder to accept pain and darkness.

We had all brought items with us, such as essential oils, seeds, dried flower petals, dried mushrooms and berries, mead — anything with a sacred or medicinal use that we knew about — some of which we would offer to the energies, some we would offer to the priestesses in thanks. At Uxmal, Merilyn told us to wear white clothes and to bring our personal offerings for the burning ceremony — a meaningful element in the ritual primicia. We would do one at the beginning at Uxmal and one at the end at Chichen Itza. The ancient Maya believed that the smoke possessed spiritual energy that carried the blessings up to the Gods.

I felt a little lost as to what to offer in gratitude. These offerings would be destroyed. Was it supposed to be something valuable? My roommate had confessed she was offering a pricey necklace, and others were also offering jewelry. I hadn't thought about anything like that. Should I offer my crystal necklace? My wedding ring? That didn't feel right and I reached further inside, searching for what piece of me I could offer wholeheartedly that still felt worthy of this sacred ceremony.

I began spending all my waking moments saying my ascension attitudes (open-eyed ascension) — my form of praying without ceasing. It brought me to a still center from which I could reflect. I found a spark of truth in thinking about offering up a painting I had made while on the journey. It had no extrinsic value, but it captured a pure moment, a moment when I was full of joy, relaxed, at ease — a moment I had wanted to preserve for myself. I worried about being judged for not leaving something with monetary value. What would it look like to the others if they left rubies and I left only a small, postcard-sized painting? Still, I decided it was right to offer what I could find of truth in myself, however small that might be.

The "why am I here?" refrain repeated itself throughout my entire journey. Every day as I was ascending I asked the question again, and watched it take me through different parts of my self and my journey. I saw that I was weaving a new story, a new legend, a new beginning. One day I wrote:

I'm here because I don't want to miss out—ostensibly not to miss out on this trip, this opportunity, but more importantly not to miss out on life. I'm here to branch out to see who I am without my roles, without my culture, without my husband and kids, but mostly so that when I return I know more of myself.
(Journal entry, December 2002)

Another day I saw:

I'm here to weave threads back to my own world. I want to know a deeper connection—to know that tickle down deep that calls me and tells me I know selfless love; I know courage; I know connection . . . I'm here to sense my own presence as part of a wind that blows everywhere as a particle and a wave.

Along with investigating why we were there and paying attention to our dreams, we were given other tasks, generally connected to different offerings we would make for the primicia. I continued to worry about my offerings and whether they were enough, but one night I had a dream in which Merilyn came to me and said, "You see, you do know." It had to do with how to do an offering. I understood then that the offering had to do with a quality in my being. It had to do with giving the best of myself.

As we were preparing for different aspects of the primicia, Merilyn told us one day that we were to go by ourselves into town the following morning and hunt for the perfect candle to represent ourselves on the altar the next day. I walked into town later, enjoying my solitude, enjoying the dusty streets and the haphazard stores so typical of Mexico. I repeated my ascension attitudes the whole time, and the experience of walking was very meditative. I asked that my candle reveal itself to me. I began looking in the stores and found many candles: tall white ones, ones in glass jars with Christian icons on them, short ones, fragrant ones, colorful ones, natural ones, but none of them seemed quite right. I kept walking, and toward the outskirts of town I saw a little store that was crammed full of stuff, something like a cross between a souvenir store, a thrift store, and an antique store. I stepped around a full coat of armor standing near the entrance and looked up at the walls covered with masks, swords, costumes, and shelves filled with stone sculptures, ceramic figurines, and leather pieces. It was a little overwhelming and certainly not a likely place to find a candle. I hesitated.

The owner saw me pause and asked, "*Que busas?*" "What are you looking for?"

"*Una vela.*" "A candle."

"*Una vela?*" he said. "*Hay velas in la tienda de comestibles.*" "There are candles in the grocery store."

"*Si pero, yo quiero una vela especial.*" "Yes, but I want a special candle." Then, "Never mind. *No importa. Gracias!*" I started to walk out.

"*Un momento, senorita,*" he called out after me. "*Ven aqui.*"

He took me by the hand and brought me to a glassed-in counter up front. There was all manner of jewelry and small figurines crammed into the dusty case.

"*Acabo de recorder que tengo una pequena vela.*" "I just remembered I have one small candle."

He unlocked the case, reached his hand down to the bottom shelf, and grasped something in his hand. It looked like it had been hidden there a long time. He pulled it out and placed it on the counter top.

"*Una vela corazon especial,*" he said. "One special heart-shaped candle."

It was exactly right.

I walked back to my room carrying my altar candle lovingly. That night I had a dream that had to do with placing items on the altar. I woke up calling, "*Mi corazon, mi corazon.*" Not only had I found my candle, I had found my heart. I would offer my heart.

* * *

We were staying in a lovely hotel right across from the ruins of Uxmal. The hotel was situated with long corridors around a central pool courtyard and dining area. In addition to our individual hotel rooms, the group had two other rooms: the hotel library, where we met each evening, and another small room, where we set up an altar and offerings. We transported this altar and the offerings from place to place, and periodically we had larger ceremonies at sacred sites. Every day we added things to the altar.

On the second day at Uxmal, I sat in the meeting room. It had been a full day of visiting the sacred site, followed by participating in a huge, ceremonial burning pile. I had ascended during most of the ceremony. It was quite remarkable being surrounded by women from all around the world, each making offerings. During our meeting that night, a feeling overcame me that all these women—all people, really—were searching for the same thing. I'd heard that before, but hadn't experienced a mixing of cultures with such a singular focus. It seemed everyone was speaking the same language, though the words were different. It made me think of the song "Love in Any Language," by Patti Smith.

That night in the group meeting, a surreal feeling overtook me and I felt almost like I was high. The edges of the room began to blur while Merilyn was talking and a great stillness—a reverence—filled the room. I looked around the room slowly at the different participants and some of them seemed to jump out at me. Their energies felt like me, but they looked different and had different personalities: Joanna, Anya, Chris. I literally saw myself in their skin. At a different time, I might have been scared by this experience, but in this moment, strangely, it felt comforting. I felt that if I had grown up in their country with their parents, my essence would have evolved just as theirs had—as if the manner in which a particular energy is squeezed is what forms it . . . I left the room at the end of the meeting feeling spacey, ungrounded, still high. Our dreaming task that night was to offer our hearts to the Ancestors, asking them to awaken and guide us.

I had trouble falling asleep, and after dozing in and out a bit, I decided to get up and walk around the beautiful grounds of the hotel. Outdoor, open-air corridors with tall columns and tile floors surrounded an interior courtyard that included a dining area and a lushly landscaped pool. The night air was warm and there was a gentle breeze that slightly rustled the lacy leaves of tall palm trees. I took my heart candle with me and paused to deliver it to the altar room. I was still feeling very odd. As I was leaving the room, I was surprised to bump into Merilyn. She turned and peered at me intently and asked sharply, "How are you?"

My response, "I am fine," was quick and instinctual—a classic, automatic Western answer.

She shivered a little and did a kind of double take at me. Then, with the most incredible scrutiny I have ever felt, she peered deeply into my eyes and said, "I said, how *are* you?"

In the next moment everything came to a complete standstill. My mind completely shut down. She was not looking for a platitude. She was looking for the truth. I felt as if I was sitting on a razor's edge. If I responded one way I would fall into one reality; if I responded another I would fall into a different reality.

On the one side was all my conditioning, everything I was used to. On the other was a complete mystery. I searched for an answer and discovered there was nothing there. She held me with her gaze. My mind teetered, went silent, and then I felt myself falling inwardly . . . to the other side.

"I . . . I don't . . . know," I said, feeling for the resonance when something rings true, and it dawned on me in that instance that the most honest thing I knew was that I didn't know anything.

What happened just afterwards was indescribable, but which different cultures have called Samadhi—transcending the bounds of the body, mind, and self-identity to merge into an undifferentiated unity with all that is.

I found myself standing in the hallway alone—Merilyn no longer standing before me. I have no idea how long I had been standing there. I had no sense of time. My attention widened, like a river overflowing its banks—spreading in all directions at once. I began walking, although it felt more like floating, toward a sound coming from a source I couldn't identify. My mind was free from the need to label my surroundings. I registered "beautiful sound," but not "song." Next, I found myself sitting in the courtyard in an ineffable state of emptiness that defied explanation. The "I don't know" state had consumed my being and left my mind undistracted and unrestricted. There was absolutely no fear present in my being. I felt like a newborn, innocent, yet curious and fresh about taking in my surroundings, but lacking any need to question or analyze. Good and bad had no reference. I was resonant with all. To the extent that there was any feeling to the moment, there was only a hint of unrepressed joy, as though I was smiling inside. I felt I was touching my own essence, and that it was shared by everyone and everything.

I have no idea how many hours I sat in that courtyard in a state of simple, unanalyzed awe—in a state of Love, without either a subject or an object. At some point, I moved back to my room.

While the Love state was not permanent, it was an inviolable experience that I will carry with me always and which colors every aspect of my life. I now knew that transcendence was possible. Still ringing with the experience, I wrote:

There have been moments in my life when the veil keeping me from seeing and experiencing myself has been lifted. My recent journey to the Yucatan with Merilyn Tunneshende afforded me one of those opportunities. This journey to the heartland of the sacred feminine with Merilyn, Maria Garcia, a Mayan priestess, Ana Maria, a woman of the heart, Miguel, a scholar of the lore of the ancient region, and with women from around the world, became for me a journey to my own heart.

I remember Merilyn asking us on the first days of the journey to consider why we were here. This eclectic group of thirty-two women ranging in age from spring chicken to winter sage, women who had come from all over the world, literally: Africa, Finland, Brazil, Russia, Europe, the United States, Mexico . . . and whose ancestries brought together even more parts of the world, had ostensibly come together to participate in an ancient ceremony, a Mayan primicia, which had not been allowed to be performed at the sacred sites of Chichen and Uxmal for over five hundred years—a ceremony which had never been open to foreigners. Yet, there we were offering ourselves to honor the occasion.

I remember turning Merilyn's question around and hearing instead "I am here. Why?" It simply dumbfounded me at some deep recess of my heart that I—a paralegal, mother, and housewife from Washington State—could find herself [sic] partaking in such a ceremony. I was inexperienced, naive, unenlightened, yet, I was there.

By the end of our journey, the "why" part of the question was disappearing and I had relaxed into the more simple "I am here." Ultimately, however, this journey to the heartland led me to the inescapable undeniable experience of "I am," and the "I" was so much bigger than I imagined, so fascinating and curious, yet completely devoid of questions, devoid of fear. I found myself in one moment completely in love with myself and even saying that cannot begin to capture the essence of that experience. It was not based on romance or desire in the least, more like I was mother to myself as a newborn baby. It was, in fact, an ineffable quality—the very resonance of life, of living, of being alive—without any box. At the time, I described this discovery as one of finding my heart to be an unplanted fertile ground. I felt myself brimming with potential—burgeoning with the essence required to bring life forth in abundance. This life I felt was not necessarily connected to the physical, but was something infinitely deeper and more mysterious, something even more compelling than physical life. I think my old heart poured out that day and became empty so that it could be filled anew. (Journal entry, January 2003)

As I came back into myself over the course of the next few days, I wanted to share my experience with Jake. I made my way through town to an international call center.

"Jake, something happened," I said, huddled in the small closet of the Mexican payphone. I struggled to find the words. "Jake—it was unbelievable. I touched infinity and there is no fear there. Everything is perfect."

"Oh, okay, I can't really talk right now; the girls have to get to gymnastics," Jake said. He sounded far away and distracted. "You can tell me all about it when you get home."

I only had a few moments to connect with him as the call was ridiculously expensive, so I turned the conversation to practical matters.

"How was the house hunting?" I asked, trying to keep the line open a bit longer. "One of the ladies here had a dream about our new house and came and told me about it."

"Interesting. Well, the kids and I had fun looking and I think we found one, but we can talk about that when you get home, too."

I could tell he wanted to go. He never loved talking on the phone.

"I miss you," I said quickly, wanting to add *and I found me.*

"Miss you too. See you in a couple days."

When I got off the phone, I wondered about the house they had found. I had told the Rainbow Women that we were moving across the country when I got home. I had explained that my husband and kids were looking at houses while I was on the journey. During the journey, one of the women came up to me and told me that she had had a dream about our new house. Really? She described in some detail the setting of what was to be our new house in North Carolina. She described a lot of sacred, forested land, a large field, and a special green rock. I couldn't help but think she was describing the ranch house and began to imagine living there. So I was very surprised when I got home to learn that Jake had put an offer on a completely different house.

"It's almost brand new in a little planned community," he said. "The kids loved it!"

I was a little taken aback. *Huh, that's weird. I really thought that woman's dream was real and that it was about the ranch house.*

"What about that ranch house?" I asked.

"Oh yeah. We saw that one too. It was a dive! It didn't help that we arrived during the worst ice storm and that all the electricity was out and two enormous trees had fallen down in the backyard. The kids hated it. It was cold, dark, and old."

"But what did *you* think?" I pestered. "It seemed like such an enchanting setting."

"Well, I thought the land was pretty cool—lots of diverse

forest up by the house and a big field and horse barn down below that I was thinking we could convert into a meditation retreat center. The decking all around the house and raised Jacuzzi deck was really neat, too. But there's a lot of work that would need to be done . . . the house was a disaster."

"So, are you still interested in it?"

"Well, since the kids loved the new house, I decided to honor their wishes and actually put an offer on that house—a good one, too—only ten thousand under the asking price."

"Huh, okay," I said, readjusting my expectations. I hadn't seen the ranch house after all—maybe I would have felt differently if I had.

Jake went on. "But in the back of my mind, I thought we could also talk to the lady with the ranch house. If she were willing to take about a hundred thousand less . . . I could be tempted."

Ten thousand under the asking price of one house? A hundred thousand under the asking price of the other? Seemed like a no-brainer—what home owner would easily accept an offer for $100,000 less than their asking price and what home owner wouldn't be willing to come down just $10,000 on their price?

As circumstances would have it, however, the owner of the almost new house absolutely refused to back off the list price, even though it had been on the market for a year and even though we only offered ten thousand dollars less. Jake was incensed.

"She won't come down at all!" he cried. "That's ridiculous!"

"Let's talk to the ranch lady," I encouraged.

So Jake and ranch lady, Susan, began corresponding. He told her all about loving the land and that if we were to get such a place, we wanted to convert the horse barn into a retreat center. He formally offered her a hundred thousand dollars less than her asking price. While they were talking back and forth, though, she got a full-price offer for the ranch house. We were surprised when she came back to us and asked us if we could come up a little.

She said, "I really want to sell it to you guys. The full-price offer is from a developer and I can't bear the thought of this beautiful property being developed."

We talked about it and decided to offer her one-third more than our previous offer. To our great surprise, she accepted.

* * *

We parked on the street and stepped under the wisteria arch. The realtor was incredibly nervous.

"You know, I have only once before shown a house to a couple who've already committed to buying it, where the wife had not seen it before. It didn't go well."

I was barely listening; I was so enchanted with the entry. Under the wisteria archway the driveway opened up. On either side grew redbuds, hickory, maple, and other big towering trees, many covered with ivy and wisteria. An old arbor covered in honeysuckle vines stood to the right. A log-cabin shed peaked from behind giant forsythia. To the left, an octagonal aviary structure could be seen, and further away, two or three more outbuildings. A wooden boardwalk picked up where the driveway left off, leading under another natural foliage archway, and curved around the short side of the rectangular rambler, whose main door faced into the forest, not the street. To the left of the boardwalk, a series of concrete steps wrapped around behind the house. Overgrown gardenias and camellias covered the end of the house, while a towering walnut tree marked the end of the boardwalk and the beginning of the decking.

"What were you saying?" I said.

"Just worried," he replied, "that you won't like it."

"Like it? I love it!" I cried.

It was like stepping into a magic cottage. The energy of the place was incredible—somehow sacred and hallowed. It turned out the land touched not only on Indian burial grounds, but also on a Baptist church and adjoining cemetery. And the forest was one of the few highly diverse pieces of forest around—the lands nearby having been logged and replanted with only pine trees. In its eclectic history, the original owners had made wilderness trails all over it, taking children and adults on nature tours to learn about all the different species of plants and trees. There were stone-lined pathways throughout the property and some of the trees still bore the little handmade wooden signs: Black Walnut, Red Mulberry, Hickory, and others. The second owners, Susan and her husband, had raised three hundred exotic birds on the land: African gray parrots, macaws, parakeets, peacocks, and many others—not to mention a tiger they had also raised for a spell until it became illegal to do so. There were two outdoor aviaries and an atrium inside the house. What was to become my office had previously been a bird nursery. The living room had floor-to-ceiling windows that looked out onto a lawn area surrounded by forest, entirely private, but with a peek-a-boo view through the trees to a single skyscraper 10 miles in the distance.

Shortly after moving in, a friend came by to live with us while he helped us build a sweat lodge on the property. He brought a gift with him: a pebble-sized piece of translucent, green obsidian that he said was rare and special and that healers told him allowed for a connection with nature and the self-realizations of love and tenderness. He placed it in the woods on a collection of boulders in the forest. It looked like green glass to me, but I couldn't help but remember the woman at the Rainbow journey who had described our new home, including a special green rock.

This was to be our sanctuary for the next eight years, and the old rambler on the big land got us through some of the sweetest— and toughest—days ever.

Chapter 27

Be Fabulous or Die

It Felt Love
How
Did the Rose
Ever open its Heart

And give to this World
All its
Beauty?

It felt the encouragement of light
Against its
Being

Otherwise,
We all remain

Too

Frightened
~ Hafiz, translated by Daniel Ladinsky

In the weeks following the move into our new house, I frequently felt like I was walking on sunshine, and would burst into the song of that name, dancing through the house, feeling light and bright, pausing to write and read poetry, trying to capture something not capturable. One day I walked into the local Barnes and Noble and headed to the poetry section where I had never been. As I reached for a book, another came out instead called *The Gift: Poems by Hafiz, The Great Sufi Master*, translated by Daniel Ladinsky. As I grabbed it, it fell open to the page with the poem "It Felt Love." It spoke to me directly. I had tasted something sweet and precious on that Rainbow journey—I too had felt the encouragement of light against my being. I felt like I was growing, evolving into the person I had always wanted to be. I was no longer seized with memories of the Petersons and felt like I had my PTSD under control.

However, at the same time that my heart had the potential to wildly expand, I was shocked to discover something missing between Jake and me. Again, Jake's work had taken a sour turn. Prior to moving across the country, and after we returned from Yelapa, Jake had found fulfilling and challenging work doing cutting-edge research for a start-up, commercially oriented engineering company. When a large, conservative, military-oriented company purchased the start-up, fired two-thirds of the workforce, and relocated the remaining workforce across the country, the new company also canceled the program Jake had been working on. Thus, almost immediately after moving, what had been satisfying work for Jake disappeared, and he was thrust again into the bowels of a big company doing military work he opposed in principle. It was not fulfilling and he did not like it. Still bearing the lion's share of responsibility in supporting our family and having agreed to be employed there for at least a year, he felt trapped once again. Plus, we were completely devoid of any supportive community. Without our extended family nearby and with the Ascension community splintered, we were also spiritually and emotionally adrift.

At this time, I didn't fully appreciate that Jake was struggling with much deeper issues that tormented him as well. He was torn once again between the two paths before him: on the one hand he had a family that was now isolated from their support structure, and who depended on him to care and provide for them; on the other hand, he had a deep yearning in his soul to know the Absolute Truth—a feeling he once described as a "splinter in my brain, constantly needling me." His divine longing came into stark relief against the backdrop of unfulfilling work conducted in an environment of colleagues who did not share his dreams of becoming enlightened. As he struggled with the splinter in his brain against the need to support his family, he turned his focus toward his desire to convert our property into a meditation retreat center—a commune, he hoped. He wanted to attract meditation teachers to our area and reasoned that if he built a retreat center, we could recreate our community where we were.

Jake felt strongly that we needed the support of a bigger community, both spiritually and to share the workload of a common piece of property. He loved the idea of being surrounded by a loving community and had long dreamed of living in a commune. In his mind's eye, he could imagine how it could be perfect—everyone sharing the same divine longing, working and playing together. Truthfully, though, Jake just worked harder than anybody else who came to help, and as they frequently were meditation teachers who had no reliable source of income, he also ended up paying them—thus increasing the number of people he was supporting and taking care of. In actuality, he had more responsibility and meditated less during this period of building a retreat. In hindsight, it is one of the things he regrets most in his life, feeling that he lost precious time with his kids pursuing that dream.

The commune idea was also often the source of fights between us. The idea didn't sit right with me. We were still in the middle of raising our kids, for one thing, who by this time were 11 and 14. I worried. What would it be like for them? What would it be like when family came to visit? Plus, I just couldn't imagine how the situation could keep from getting sticky. It scared me.

When he talked about it, I interpreted it as meaning that he was not committed to us. I began to micro-examine his actions and, while he never said as much, I often inferred that he didn't really want me, that he was judging me and found me lacking.

At the same time, while our property was enchanting and beautiful, it was also a pile of work, and we were always busy with yard labor. It is not work that I excelled at, and I frequently felt like I failed in his eyes. Jake is a natural and tireless, loving gardener and landscaper. He can envision what something could look like and knows just what to do to get there; he can work for an entire day doing hard labor. He brings an attitude of reverence to the plants and critters that share the land. While he cleaned, leveled, and shaped our property with enthusiasm, he never did so heedlessly, agonizing over which trees might need to be cut down and whether he was destroying any habitats, even allowing the copperheads to co-exist on our property. I, on the other hand, didn't have the vision, the natural affinity, or physical endurance to match his pace. When he left for work, he would leave me detailed instructions as to what to get done and always I would get less done than he hoped. I began to mentally tally all the ways that I had not lived up to his expectations.

I began to tally other things too. *When was the last time he said "I love you"?* When I approached him and wrapped my arms around his neck, he had developed a habit of putting his hands on his hips, not engaging my affection. *When was the last time he approached me on his own?* I added to the tally. There was a huge space growing between us and, ultimately—despite all the sunshine I was walking on—I found our lack of intimacy terrifying and confusing. At some point—possibly because he was doing so much physical construction work on the barn conversion, possibly because the whole idea of marriage was something of an anathema to him at the time—he stopped wearing his wedding ring—on which was inscribed the words "sharing dreams." I began to realize that we were not really sharing dreams any longer. In some ways, we were not really acting like a "we" at all—a thought I had never considered—a thought that stupefied my mind because of its potential to blow up all the boundaries that I thought kept me safe, kept me loved.

One day, I realized that as good as our sex was, our lovemaking had lost its deeper connection; we could still be intensely physical and play wild sex games with each other, but it felt like we were no longer truly intimate with one another. Somewhere along the way, despite our training, we had lost the sacred part of sacred sex and I found our connection hollow.

When I saw it, I was shocked. Everything inside me rebelled. Suddenly, I didn't care about enlightenment or the huge expansion I had experienced; all I wanted was intimacy. I wanted reciprocated love. I wanted reciprocated commitment.

Our old patterns began to repeat themselves. I got clingy and needy, and he withdrew, angry and uncommunicative. My feeling of walking on sunshine disappeared into a feeling of despair.

In my journal I wrote:

We had just moved across the country. I was at once excited and terrified, energized and exhausted . . . I was needy and independent, stable and unstable . . . I felt like I was plutonium itself filled with potential, yet desperately unstable under certain conditions.
(Journal entry, February 2003)

When those conditions surfaced, my fearful, rational mind took over and shut out the mystical. It's all well and good to seek enlightenment, but what about us! My unhealthy attachment to Jake—the one Merilyn Tunneshende had tried to warn me about—reared its head and sent me into my second dark night of the soul, much like the first one when I called the crisis hotline, and like it, triggered feelings of abandonment and insecurity—

the heart of my karmic conditioning.

One night in particular, Jake was depressed, angry, and shut down, and despite my repeated attempts to draw him out and to get him to talk to me, he was having none of it. There was nothing I could do to reach him. I felt helpless.

"Jake, I want to help you," I pleaded.

"Go away, Mariah. Leave me alone. Go figure out your own life. I just want to go to sleep!"

"Where should I go?" I pestered. "What should I do?"

Jake, wrapped up in his own misery, yelled back "I don't care! I can't help you, and I don't want to. You can't help me. I'm a tormented soul. You keep trying to cheer me up. I don't want to be cheered up. I don't need you. Leave me alone, and let me be."

Cold, biting, painful words. His eyes held no warmth, his pupils constricted. He was in his own world fighting his own demons, closed to me. Jake and I were on different trajectories at this point and we each needed to run our own separate course. Essentially we each had to enter into the dark night alone. I could no more understand his path than he could understand mine.

I looked at him, and drenched in self-pity, felt utterly rejected all over again. All my fears were true. He doesn't need me. He doesn't want me. I am unlovable and unworthy. I grabbed my jacket and cell phone and ran out of the house in pure flight mode. I ran crazily and haphazardly into the pitch-black winter night, into the forest—over stumps and dead branches, through low-growing bushes under towering trees—until I collapsed on the ground sobbing. All my fears and insecurities came back with a vengeance, starting with the singular thought: *I am on my own.* And with that thought I simply wailed into the night. A mantra of related thoughts screamed inside my head: *I don't want to be alone. I can't be alone. I can't live without Jake. I don't want to.*

Lying in the dark huddled under my jacket, clutching my cell phone, suffering viscerally, the hours slipped by. I stared at my phone, knowing I needed help, and wondered whether I should call somebody, but I didn't feel like talking to anyone. My thoughts were despairing. *I can't do this. I can't do life. Nobody can help me. I need him . . . but he doesn't need me. I want to die.* And with that thought a whole new cycle of vicious thoughts took over and the tone changed. The voice in my head, which sounded remarkably like me, was now mean and judging, but terribly convincing.

That's right, it would be better to just die. If Jake doesn't want to be with you, then you should just go ahead and die. It's not worth living. You've done everything and you've failed. You will never get it right. You've tried diving into your fears and exposing all your vulnerabilities, and yet here you are, broken again. You say you've touched god, and yet here you are, still unworthy, still unlovable, still not enough. The litany went on unchecked.

The night was getting colder. *Maybe I will freeze. Maybe I will fall asleep and never wake up.* I began to imagine my body actually dying—my light going out permanently. It might be peaceful to just slowly fade away into the dark. The way I was living right now was a slow death, anyway. I imagined everybody's life after my death. The kids would recover; Jake would find someone else, or perhaps start a commune that actually worked. Life would be better without me.

The dark began giving way to dawn. I had been out in the freezing woods all night long, wanting to die. Maybe I would just take some pills. I shivered under my jacket, miserable. I thought about Jake inside, warm and cozy. He didn't even come looking for me!

A bird began singing in those wee hours and my attention wandered from my own suffering to listen for a moment. The sound was so pure, so sweet, so beautiful. It made me smile despite myself. As I listened, a thought occurred to me: Where did that sound come from? It just revealed itself, I realized. I had nothing to do with it. And while it was natural for a bird to start singing in the morning, it was not something I could will to happen. I had no control over it whatsoever.

The morning rays began filtering through the trees, bringing the forest and me into the light. I was near the place where the green rock rested on the boulders. Wait . . . wait . . . Something deep inside myself called out . . . wait a minute . . . I felt a shift inside as I paused from my self-hatred for one long moment. Something was off. And then there it was. I saw the flaw in my plan to die. I may not love myself or find myself worthy of living . . . but I *love* life itself! Appreciation and gratitude rushed through me.

Whether life needs me or not, whether I am worthy or not, I love it. I love its simplicity. I love how the sun rises quietly, bringing light to a dark world. I love how the birds start singing. I love how the sun sets, allowing time for rest. I love the feel of grass beneath my feet and the scent of wisteria on the air. I love the way that tree grows crookedly up between other trees as it seeks light. I love when it rains quietly *and* when it pours wildly. I love laughing joyously. I love crying freely. I love being alive! I get to be alive! I am alive! I cannot control life. It just is.

Something inside me broke free as I realized that my love of Life was not conditioned on anything after all. Life doesn't have to prove itself worthy; it just is. Life doesn't have to be perfect to be loved. And neither do I.

Still huddled on the ground, my face cold and wet, I surrendered finally to the understanding that Life—much as I wanted it to be, much as I felt responsible for it to be—was simply not under my control any more than the planes that once terrified me. I wanted to get up and shout to the world: Life! It's beautiful just the way it is. I felt my commitment then to keep living, to keep loving, but to let go of the root agreement I had seen that first night of the dreaming workshop: my attachment to death. I let go of, too—not my love, not my commitment—but my unhealthy attachment to Jake.

I saw something else too. I saw how important it is to live life fully in all its imperfect, crooked, happy, sad glory—and that to do anything less than to love fearlessly without the need to control or be controlled by another was to die a slow death, anyway. With that came words I was to live by: Be Fabulous or Die.

* * *

It was strange filtering back into my life after the night in the woods. From outward appearances everything was the same, but I was not the same. I felt the need to honor and accept Jake and our relationship exactly where he was and where it was.

"Jake," I said, approaching him some days later in our bedroom, "I know you have already taken off your wedding ring, and you told me once you didn't want to be married per se. Here," I said, handing him my wedding ring. He looked strangely—inscrutably—at me. I couldn't really tell what he was thinking and he didn't offer up much.

"Huh. Well, okay. Let's just put them here on our altar."

The symbolic gesture didn't take much time. We were each on our own now. Together physically still, raising a family still, but detached.

I decided to become a certified mediator and start my own mediation business, in addition to my ongoing freelance paralegal work. It took a lot of focus to try to start that business from scratch but I greatly enjoyed volunteering at the Durham courthouse to gain the necessary experience required by the state. Eventually, I became one of the few certified non-attorney mediators in North Carolina. Unfortunately I never did make a lot of money at it.

One day during this time, as an act of pure independence, I spontaneously bid on a car auction on eBay. It's something Jake would never have done. It was in the early days of eBay and I didn't perfectly understand the ramifications at the time, but my sister-in-law, who was visiting, raved about how great it was and how she had just bought a new bike using eBay. I decided to look at the cars online. I squealed when I saw a somewhat affordable, gorgeous purple Volkswagen bug. Before I fully appreciated what I was doing, I discovered I had "won" the auction. Oops. Normally, Jake would have handled the financial end of things like that, but as I had obviously been making a statement of independence, I knew I had to take care of all the details myself. I took myself down to the bank and figured out how to get a loan. Then I discovered that the car I had just purchased was located in Texas! Oops again and ouch. To his credit Jake said very little, perhaps wondering silently how I was going to solve that little snafu . . . But I did solve it by paying Durga to take a bus out to Texas to pick it up and drive it back. When it arrived I discovered that it was even more beautiful than the pictures, because its iridescent paint shifted between shades of purple and dark blue in different lights—kind of psychedelic. I loved that car. But truthfully, it was a lemon. In less than a year the engine seized, and when I went to all the trouble to get another one for it, that one died a couple months later too. Sigh. It was all a sort of huge mistake, but it was one I made on my own.

The whole thing sounds ridiculous, but in some way both the mediating work and the VW bug were important steps for me. Strangely enough, the journal entries that I had written during the Vashon Island dream retreat with Merilyn mention dreams featuring both "mediating" (which, at the time, I had interpreted as "meditating") and "a purple swirly psychedelic cover for a slug bug car." Those dreams, it turned out, were divine winks foreshadowing what was to come: important baby steps to my "be fabulous or die" insight.

Chapter 28

Meanwhile, Back at the Ranch

Just keep swimming, swimming, swimming.
~ Dory in *Finding Nemo*

Meanwhile, back at the ranch, Jake kept building the converted-barn retreat center over the course of the year—pushing himself to extremes, working for hours after coming home from work, and on the weekend. We had invited meditation teacher-friends to come and help us build. I no longer resisted his work and enjoyed the company of the people we had helping us. Maybe a commune wasn't such a bad idea, after all.

It was difficult for Jake, however, because many of the meditation teachers who came to help did not have any money or even any livelihoods, so in order to get them to help, we had to offer them a place to live and/or a wage. Thus, it wasn't truly a joint and balanced venture. It was our land and Jake's hard-earned money supporting the entire endeavor. This made it difficult for Jake because he had envisioned cocreating a meditation retreat center, but he was single-handedly funding it. Jake felt like he ended up with most of the responsibility and that he worked twice as hard as anyone else.

At the same time, around the fall of 2003, Jake's dad got sick with lung cancer. It was the second time he'd had cancer, having battled throat cancer some years earlier. We thought he would beat the cancer this time, too. Still, it pained Jake to live so far away while his dad was sick, but he felt it was impossible to change the situation. We couldn't afford to move back. The job situation in Seattle in his field was still dicey. If we left, we'd have to reimburse the company for all the moving expenses, plus incur new ones, and because Jake hadn't worked here a year yet, he would also lose his stock options. Moving back would cost over a hundred thousand dollars with no guarantee of employment on the other side.

At the end of the year, Jake went on the men's retreat with Merilyn Tunneshende. She had told me once that we would be the only couple to both complete the training. At the time she told me, I thought it was important, but by the time he went, I ascribed no great significance to the fact. Jake came back with his own lessons from the journey, having been pushed to his physical limits of endurance while participating in a ritual sweat. "I saw that my pride would kill me," he said upon returning. "It was an important lesson."

"What happened?" I asked.

"We did a native sweat ritual which was made up of three 45-minute sweats. We were told that we could leave if we wanted to, but I found I couldn't leave in front of the others. The sweat was unbearably hot, and after the first 45 minutes I couldn't stand it. All the men, in fact, were lying on the ground moaning, and obviously suffering."

"Did anybody leave?"

"No. But I saw that I should have. It was dangerous. They opened the door to let some fresh air in between sessions and I could have left, but couldn't bring myself to go. We did a second session and it was pure torture. From one moment to the next I simply endured, giving myself up to the possibility of dying. I literally saw that I would rather die than lose face by leaving earlier than others."

The lesson, as valuable as it was, did not bring Jake peace. And as 2004 began, Jake continued to be depressed. He was deeply conflicted about what to do with his life. He felt completely in limbo and struggled on many fronts. He felt bad about taking the kids away from their family and friends, about not living closer to his mom and dad while his dad was sick. He was disappointed in his job, and he still wanted to start a spiritual community and meditate more. He wasn't sure if I still shared his dreams and where we were headed together. As often happens when people are depressed, he couldn't remember any of our good times — he simply couldn't remember them — and so he replayed our struggles over and over.

In April, a little over a year after we had moved to North Carolina, he decided he had to do something drastic. He requested a three-month leave from work, but this was denied, so he quit, leaving his well-paying job and all its benefits. He wrote up a plan where we would live extremely frugally on one quarter of his previous income per year, but still he was not happy. I watched him slip into an even deeper depression and from my new — detached — vantage point, did my best not to interfere any longer. One day I came in and found him lying on the couch watching the movie *Kill Bill*. This was not that worrisome until he watched it four more times in a row.

Then Jake announced he wanted to do a sweat. I agreed, as did our friend, Durga, who was staying with us. It seemed like a good idea to mark his new beginning. He wanted something to shift, something that would propel him forward again.

The sweat lodge we had built on our land comprised a round circle made up of huge logs standing on end. The inside of the circle was lined in thick canvas, which also draped across the top of the logs to form a low ceiling — too low to stand in, but big enough to sit in. Long poles, draped in a tarp, formed a water-proof, teepee-style cover over the whole structure. Inside, a deep pit lined in stones sat in the center. A doorway faced east to an outdoor fire pit filled with rocks we had found on the land. These were the size of two fists, perfect for a sweat.

We took our sweats seriously and entered them with

241

reverence and ritual. We prepared for them during the day, drinking extra water, limiting coffee intake, and staying completely away from alcohol. Jake was the fire tender, and on sweat days he'd start the fire hours early to allow the rocks time to heat up. We would enter the sweat clockwise, saying the traditional words, "All my relations," and proceed to our spots. He would be the last to enter, first adding hot rocks via pitchfork to the interior pit. After he entered, and in keeping with native sweat-lodge practice, he would say a kind of prayer honoring the four directions, then offer some copal and anoint the rocks with water to start the sweat. We tended to sweat twice, the first for about 20 minutes after which we'd go outside and cool off, and then go in again for one more, usually shorter, sweat. We brought plenty of water to drink, mindful of the dangers of dehydration.

On this day, however, Jake acted out of character. In the first place, he drank plenty of coffee rather than water. Then when he went to make the fire, he announced that we had to make this the hottest sweat ever. He said he wanted to stay in it longer and do three rounds instead of two.

Once we got inside, Jake brought in the rocks—nine of the largest he could find, compared to the five or seven medium-sized ones we usually started with. As he clambered in and shut the door, he quickly poured water on the rocks, foregoing all ritual. Durga and I stayed in as long as we could, but left the first sweat before him. He repeated the process two more times, and Durga joined him though didn't stay in as long; I declined to return the third time, as I was spent.

Jake was pacing like a tiger after the sweat—kind of manic in a way. He suggested we sit around the fire for a while. I was surprised when he got himself a glass of wine, unheard of on sweat day, but said nothing. Clearly he was pushing the limits, but that was his tendency and choice. He was on his own path. Later, we watched a movie. Jake drank another glass of wine, and then made himself a cup of tea before heading to bed. I found out the next day it was detox tea, which is supposed to help rid the body of toxins but which can also increase dehydration and is supposed to be taken with plenty of water—stupid, stupid, stupid.

I was awakened in the middle of the night by Jake calling my name.

"Mariah," he said, "I've got the worst headache in the world. I think you need to take me to the hospital."

I immediately woke up entirely. Jake was asking to go to the hospital? He hates doctors, doesn't trust the medical community. Normally, I am the one pestering him to go to the doctor, but this time I felt uneasy about it. It didn't seem like a good idea to jump into the car and rush to the hospital. The hospital was 20 minutes away.

"Jake," I whispered back, "you are probably dehydrated. Let me get you some water or Pedialyte. And then I'll call the hospital."

I got up quickly and decided I should wake Durga. I had the feeling this also was a spiritual crisis for Jake and that Durga might be able to help him. I ran downstairs.

"Durga, wake up—Jake is in crisis, says he has the worst headache ever. He wants me to take him to the hospital, but I think we should call 911 instead. Will you sit with him while I find the Pedialyte and call?"

She immediately went to sit with him and tried to distract his attention away from the excruciating pain. She got him up and brought him into the living room in case we had to go. Meanwhile, I found the Pedialyte, gave it to him, and dashed into my office to call 911. I could hear some noises from the living room just outside my door. Jake had swigged the Pedialyte, then gotten up and was staggering.

"I think I'm going to throw up," I heard him say.

The operator picked up. "Hello, what is your emergency?"

I heard a noise in the background and took the phone with me to look. Jake had fallen into a chair. He was absolutely white. Durga was standing near him.

"My husband has a terrible headache," I told the operator. "He says it's the worst one he's ever had. We need an ambulance!"

"Mariah!" Durga screamed from the other room. "Jake's not breathing."

"Oh my God, oh my God!" I ran into the living room holding the phone, telling the operator "My husband's not breathing. How fast can you get here?" I knelt in front of Jake. He still wasn't breathing.

"Ten to fifteen minutes," the operator said.

"Fifteen minutes!" I screamed. "He'll be dead in fifteen minutes. What do I do?"

At that moment, Jake's body jerked, then he coughed, threw up a little, and started breathing again, very shallowly.

"Wait, wait a second," I said into the phone. "I think he's breathing again. Can you hang on?" I dropped the phone without waiting to hear the response, grabbed his head and said, "Jake, are you there? Jake, come back. Come back."

He fluttered his eyelids a bit and seemed to try to open them for a minute, but he wasn't focusing on anything. His skin and even his lips were the color of a sheet of paper. I have never seen anything like that.

Meanwhile, Durga had run outside to meet the ambulance on the street, because it was hard to see our driveway.

I picked up the phone. "He's breathing a little," I told the operator.

"Okay, just calm down. The ambulance will be there in a few minutes."

I sat there kneeling before him for some minutes more, whispering to him to hang in there. But he stopped breathing again.

"He stopped breathing again!" I cried into the phone.

"Is he in a seated position?" the operator asked.

"Yes, yes . . . Jake, Jake wake up . . . don't die."

"Stay with me," the operator commanded. "I want you to get him out of the chair so that he is lying flat on the floor."

I grabbed Jake under the arms and pulled him off the chair to the ground. He coughed again and once again started breathing. I held him in my arms.

I heard noises outside and realized that the ambulance had arrived in less than 15 minutes. Within moments, the paramedics were inside taking his blood pressure and starting an intravenous drip.

The medic turned to me and said, "We can't move him for a while. His blood pressure is the lowest I have ever recorded."

The IV fluids and some sort of internal deep will to survive brought Jake back to life. He told us later that he knew he was dying—that everything went pitch black and became very peaceful. He felt like he was sinking into the blackness, and wanted to give in to it, but a thought occurred to him that he hadn't finished raising his daughters, so he struggled back to the surface, to the light.

With blood pressure of 60/30, Jake almost didn't make it back. If I had driven him to the hospital myself, he wouldn't have made it. By the time we actually did get to the hospital, the crisis was over, and the stay was uneventful. We went to the hospital just to be on the safe side, but were able to return home after a few hours. The fluids that the paramedics administered at our house had brought Jake back to life and physically into balance again. Coming into emotional balance, however, would still take some work.

"You should go and see Krishnananda, Jake," Durga urged. "It's a tight little community up there in Salmon Arm, Canada; something powerful is happening."

Jake had not fully bounced back after his near death experience.

"I don't know what to do," he confessed. "I am miserable. I feel like misery is my path."

The three of us had been talking about options and Durga had strongly urged him to go away on retreat for a month—anything would be better than sitting on the couch watching endless reruns of *Kill Bill*, she reasoned.

Krishnananda, one of the Ascension teachers, had broken off and started a new organization in Canada. We had heard through the grapevine that some people thought he was great—an enlightened teacher. One of Jake's heartfelt desires at this time was to find a teacher to guide him. He decided to go.

Jake would be gone over his birthday and totally unreachable. I yearned to connect with him, to talk to him, to tell him everything would be okay, but there was still a distance between us. I also knew that I had to honor my own fledgling self, who had spread her wings of independence, remaining committed, but not attached to the outcome. I had to trust that he would work it all out on his own, as I had.

Afterward, Jake told me that when he first arrived at the retreat, he felt like his heart was almost completely shut down. He said he felt totally alone and adrift. He spent the first days there angry and rebellious. Because there had been such finger pointing during the break-up of the Ascension community, he didn't know whom to trust. He was reluctant to open up. One night in the meeting, he stood up and directly challenged Krishnananda by asking him point blank if he was enlightened. Krishnananda answered that he experienced "endless peace."

The next morning was Jake's birthday. He had gotten into a routine of walking in the morning with a group of Mexican participants, who found out it was his birthday. At the retreat, it was customary for all the participants, who had come from around the world, to sing "Happy Birthday" in all the different versions that each country had to offer. When they sang to him, Jake said he experienced a flood of love, and that it opened his heart.

Back at home, I wrote a letter in my journal to him on his birthday, just for myself:

Jake,

I am thinking of you. I know it seems dark and I know you have the will to live and to find the light. You showed me, so I'll stop worrying. If you are struggling right now, you must need to. I know this battle is real to you. I want to talk to you about sweet, gentle moments in life, about the many times we laid together and said little, how you taught me to listen. I'd wait and wait as still as I could because sometimes you'd start talking in the quiet contemplative way you had—the words sounded almost like music, like your gentle voice when you sing—so resonant and unique, like your smell.

You, dearest one, are not so strong as you think.

Please be gentle with yourself. Remember what you love about yourself—about life; remember your feminine side. Maybe, dear one, something is all wrong, and that's ok. Maybe you've been trying to prove something all along that's fundamentally false.

Right now, I realize to be afraid of you not being with me is selfish. I will be ok; the kids will be ok; you will be ok. Maybe being also afraid that you want to be with me is selfish too. Maybe we just let things unfold and see what happens. All I know right now is I want to wish you a Happy Birthday. Maybe, dear one, you do not have to be the tormented soul. Maybe you can just be happy. Work a little. Play a little. Laugh a little. (We have to work on that one.) Cry a little. Love a little.

Maybe sex is like breathing and we can just go ahead and fuck like rabbits because it is fun. Maybe sex is not that important at all. The point is Jake—I do hope you find your way and that Grace prevails for you. I do know that just because I can't see or know something doesn't mean anything. Life is a mystery—there are lots of playmates. Who are you? What do you like to play?

Happy Birthday. Remember music and dancing. Remember open-air markets and the quest for garlic soup and coconuts. Remember long walks hand in hand. Remember another girl who thought you were so sexy she had to sleep with you.

I think, my dear, you have more to do. My role is unclear, but I trust I can walk through one step at a time.

(Journal entry, 10 May 2004)

Jake said that something shifted for him following the birthday song experience, and love flooded back in. He wrote in his own journal that day:

I feel very funny, very sore & tired & dizzy. I feel like I'm almost done. I love you Mariah. I love you Jacki. I love you Cassie. I love you Durga. Thank you guys for spending time with me, for your love. I love you Jake.

The next day at the meeting, Jake said, everything was a blur. All of a sudden he found himself standing before the group, opening his mouth and asking Krishnananda to be his teacher. There is natural trepidation in asking for a formal teacher, because it is presumed that you will do whatever they say in order to gain more peace. There is a typical fear that you will be asked to do things you might not be comfortable doing. There is a fear that you may be asked to walk through suffering to get to a better place. Jake said he was prepared for that, but describes that Krishnananda took a different track in questioning his resolve. Jake said that Krishnananda repeatedly asked him, "Will you not judge how it looks? Will you do what I say?"

"Absolutely," Jake responded.

Krishnananda paused, and before agreeing to be his teacher, asked finally, "Will you walk through happiness?"

Such a notion that is—surrendering to happiness . . .

"Yes," Jake said, "I will."

Krishnananda advised him to take white novitiate vows— dedicating himself to purity and joy and evolving consciousness. At the ceremony, he was given the name "Rudra," a variation of Shiva, the Hindu god of destruction and restoration.

That night in the dorm room of the retreat center, he said a flooding of thousands of memories came back to him about all the wonderful moments we had shared. He wrote pages and pages in his journal documenting this. In the morning, he asked Krishnananda if he could go home. Krishnananda consented and said he did not have to do anything special other than to check in periodically, and to come back from time to time for an extended retreat.

A week later, Jake came home early. He called and said something marvelous had happened. He said he had a surprise.

I met him at the airport, somehow nervous to see this man I had known and lived with for over 20 years. What was this surprise? Was he finally going to become a monk? Finally going to go to teacher training? Was he joining the Ascension community? We got in the car, but before we got home, he asked me to pull over on a side road. My thoughts went back to another time long ago, when we had pulled over on a side road and he had told me his truth.

"Let's get out of the car," he said and pulled me into his arms. "Look, it's a beautiful moon and starlit night." We gazed upward together for a minute. I hadn't felt his arms around me like that in a long while.

He dropped down to his knees and gazed up at me, holding me in a deep, loving gaze.

"Mariah, will you marry me . . . again? It can be a mystical union this time."

I was stunned. I had not even remotely been expecting this surprise.

I gave him a sidewise look, thinking I could just say yes and be done. But after all we had been through . . . I looked back at him with a sparkle in my own eyes. "You are going to have to court me first."

He smiled, stood up, and said with conviction, "You are worth it. I'd be honored." Durga once told me Rudra was a man of few words but he made them count. These melted my heart. *You are worth it too*, I thought. He gathered me into his arms and held me tight.

We decided to honor our original wedding date, and a couple of months later, we took off on an extended road trip throughout the southeast to celebrate our new and twentieth wedding anniversary. A friend had offered to officiate at our private ceremony on Dauphin Island, Alabama, at the Shell Mound Indian Park —an historical site of some spiritual significance in that it is the 3000-year-old burial grounds for the Yagnahoula, or holy women of the Nahoula tribe. We exchanged new vows and old rings under an 800-year-old oak tree in the park, before heading to the French Quarter of New Orleans—the site of our tenth anniversary. We stayed in the same place on Toulouse Street as we had stayed then, Miss Anna's Creole Cottage at the Olivier House Hotel.

Later that year, Jake made plans to visit his meditation teacher and to go on retreat for a week. We couldn't both go away for the whole time because of the kids' schedules, but he suggested that I meet him there to overlap for a couple of days, which we could manage. He wanted me to experience the new community and Krishnananda. A funny feeling overcame me once I was there and I asked if I could stay on for a bit, while he went home to take care of the children. I met with Krishnananda and told him about my experience in Mexico. I said that I wanted to keep growing, but that I didn't want to lose my connection to that particular experience. He told me you can never lose what you have gained.

I also decided to take novitiate vows; mine were red, which meant I was dedicated to a path of unconditional love. I received a spiritual name too: Prema, which means "love" in Sanskrit and Hindi. Krishnananda said that, when embodied, Prema means Goddess of Divine Love, Supreme Love, Unconditional Love, and Love of the Divine Mother. I liked that. Like Venus, who had appeared so long ago in Jake's dream, I too am a goddess of Love.

* * *

As we neared the end of 2004, we had new names, and renewed commitments to each other and to the Path. Equally important, we also committed to finding balance in all of our life. Jake had seen that spending time with his kids and me was as important to him as working in the world. He backed off on the dream to build and run a retreat center—in the end he found the Universe had not supported it. Instead of it unfolding joyfully, it had been a time and money sinkhole that increased his stress. He found ways to weave his and our dreams together. He started his own consulting business and almost immediately started working for a well-backed start-up company doing cutting-edge commercial (not military) work in his field. Traditionally, start-ups threaten to take up as much time as you will give, but in this regard, Jake was stalwart. He explained from the start he would have to take off extended time to go on family vacations and meditation retreats several times per year.

A few months after Jake started working for the start-up company, the Universe had another surprise for us, when the company hired me to work as a consultant. Jake had encouraged me to apply. They needed a buyer/negotiator and were excited, he said, to hear about my mediation background—funny how things work out. Now we could both contribute to supporting the family. As it turns out, we were also able to invite Durga to live with us and help take care of our youngest daughter, who was still living at home, enabling us to travel for work when needed.

We got over the car fiasco too and one day, on a whim, Jake replaced it with a used sky-blue convertible with a personal license plate: SkyDancer.

For the next many years, Jake and I worked together for the same company, working hard, but taking care to always take time out to play with the kids, taking them to swim with the dolphins in Bimini, to see the Mayan ruins of the Yucatan, to Europe and Puerto Rico. And between those trips to be sure that we meditated and practiced sacred sexuality regularly, and that we got away together for meditation retreats at least once, often twice a year.

We had learned that our conscious choices could keep me from falling into anxiety and worry, keep Jake from slipping into depression and feeling trapped, and ultimately lead us home to our own inviolable cores side-by-side on a journey to More together.

Epilogue: Mystical Union

"SkyDancing": floating beyond the physical body, into the universe of pure energy and pure consciousness . . .
~ Margot Anand

The scent of mountain chaparral perfumed the air as we walked up the trail. The moonscape desert scene of giant rounded boulders and dusty hills that make up the Owens Valley, near Lone Pine, California, shimmered behind us. We had just completed a five-day silent meditation retreat and were making our way up to the "Ashrama," as the locals called it: a stone church built in the shape of an equilateral cross, high in the Sierras, close to Mt Whitney. We were carrying overnight packs and breathing heavily, pausing often to rest on our trek up the mountain and to take in the crisp beauty. Franklin Merrell-Wolff, a mathematician, mystic and philosopher, had built the Ashrama, which means "spiritual meeting place," some 80 years earlier. The Ashrama was a summer school for his students, who helped build it; each stone hand-placed. Although he never completed his Harvard doctorate, his followers referred to him as Dr Wolff or "Yogi." Dr Wolff always said that anyone who found the way to his door would find the door open. He died at age 98, the year after we were married, long before we had turned our own attention to the pursuit of higher consciousness. Eventually though, we aspired to walk the mystic's path, and Dr Wolff's writings profoundly moved us. So, on this day, our twenty-fifth anniversary, we found our way to his home and to his Ashrama. The door was still open.

On the cold cement floor we built a love nest in the west wing, cushioned with our pads and sleeping bags and a colorful batik sarong from Costa Rica. As we had learned years ago during love and ecstasy training at the SkyDancing Tantra Institute, we blessed the space and each other, then got undressed like new lovers, almost giggling at each other, we felt such light-hearted enjoyment at that moment. These bodies that we had ravished in all the least conventional ways for going on 28 years were still titillated at the sight of one another. With nothing but the mountains and each other as witness, we traipsed naked around the interior of the stone church, pausing to look out the windows at the high sierra beauty. As we lay down together, our dance of intimacy began.

I drew him into my mouth and all the way down my throat. As the juices began to flow, we switched positions so that we could soul gaze while he massaged my yoni and worked to insert his hand inside me, a position that I loved, but one that was laced with vulnerability and required deep trust. Long ago, we had deliberately sought out each nodule of tension inside my vagina—nodules that held memories, nodules that held shame—and long ago released them, leaving my vaginal tissue awake and vibrant, pulsing.

I pumped him steadily, varying my stroke and the placement of my hand just so. I kept my other hand moving gently over his testicles at the same time. I had learned over the course of many years and intimate communications that this greatly increased and extended his pleasure. There was a feeling of rendering of flesh before he got all the way inside. I screamed in abandonment, and ultimate surrender, as we entered this realm together. He whispered, "Pump me faster," holding my gaze when I faltered, and that brought my attention back to the moment, to an indelible connection with another being, with him, with the Universe.

At some point, the energy shifted away from the primal need for release and into a timeless space of communion—of mystical union. As we soul gazed, we breathed and moved together, as we had learned long ago. Riding the wave of bliss, as Margot had called it, everything slowed and stilled. The air felt electric, surreal. Feelings were unbounded. Passion arose in waves of ecstasy, as our hearts melted and melded, beyond the body, beyond all thoughts, beyond all previous baggage, all history. There was no fear in that space of stillness. There was nothing lacking, no needs or wants, only unbridled acceptance of each other . . . and perfect presence.

We made love for hours, taking small breaks in between where we ran naked outside the church to drink in the stark beauty of the mountains. We laughed and played like children. God, whatever or whoever that is, was certainly present.

Eventually, we gave way to release. He and I climaxed in close proximity. My yoni came, unleashing clitoral pleasure but, as frequently happened when we made love, the more powerful part of my orgasm started near my belly and worked its way up my entire body, unleashing a further river of bliss, my tears a sure sign that the energy had passed through my heart. We came laughing, joyful. We felt as close to one as two can get.

Afterward, in closing and as a way to transition back to everyday life, we stood in front of one another, closed our eyes and bowed our heads, as we had after almost every lovemaking session for the last 13 years. After standing still for a breath or two, we brought our palms together in prayer position touching one another lightly, raised our heads, and gazed once again deep into each other's eyes, then said simultaneously, "I honor you . . . as an aspect of Myself."

Afterword

Almost 18 years after the events that precipitated our journey, I have the benefit of hindsight. I now know that a journey such as this does not have a definitive end. It is ongoing.

It is my own commitment to keep practicing what I've learned, what brings me back to center, what allows the possibility of mystical union with my beloved, and what reminds me that I have a choice: Be Fabulous or Die.

In the years since, I have learned firsthand that just as you can rewire your brain to experience more peace, fewer PTSD episodes, and less depression through regular meditation, so, too, you can rewire it back to suffering. Finding the Way and getting "more" out of life each day requires an ongoing willingness to surrender in every moment to what is. Practicing sacred sexuality with my husband keeps us connected to each other, while committing to a practice of meditation keeps me connected to my own core, as does approaching life with a hint of curiosity, and a generous serving of acceptance. Sometimes I fail. I accept that too, because the sooner I do, the sooner I return to delight in the sheer experience of living.

After writing this memoir, I contacted Margot Anand to thank her for her role in my own healing—to let her know that she opened the door to recovery from sexual trauma for me—that she opened the door to "more" for me. I wanted to let her know that to this day, 18 years later, I practice the things she taught us during that yearlong Love and Ecstasy Training. I told her that her sexual healing practices, along with regular meditation, played a fundamental role in helping me to let go of the past, to let go of shame, to heal, to overcome the potential "victim" identity that threatened to consume me, and ultimately led me to experience my full potential in life and living again. I told her that I was grateful, too, that this path allowed my husband and I to experience connection and intimacy again—to be vulnerable with one another—to trust.

As you might imagine, writing this memoir was also a personal journey for me, and it wasn't until I reached out to Margot Anand after completing it that I fully appreciated how important these practices are to others. Margot not only encouraged me to get the book published, but also made a point of bringing my attention back to the suffering that still exists in the world. Having dedicated her own life to sexual healing, she knows its potential and is passionate about sharing it. She talked to me about the horrors in other parts of the world where women and girls are still exploited in the global commercial sex trade. She talked to me about cultures where there are still laws that require an underage female rape victim to marry the rapist, and how some women kill themselves rather than do so.

As I reflected on her words, I decided to look up statistics about sexual abuse here at home in the US. I was shocked by what I read. Women Organized Against Rape (WOAR), reports the following:

• 1 in 3 American women will be sexually abused during their lifetime. (George Mason University, Worldwide Sexual Assault Statistics, 2005)

• 1 in 4 women and 1 in 6 men will be sexually assaulted before the age of 18. (Finkelhor et al., 1990)

• Every 2 minutes someone somewhere in America is sexually violated. (www.rainn.org)

And while, of course, I had heard about abuse by church elders, I had never fully appreciated those statistics either. On a site called bishop-accountability.org I read that "Over 3,000 civil lawsuits have been filed in the United States between 1984 and

2009" against the Catholic Church for sexual abuse, particularly of young boys, and that it is estimated that more than 100,000 children have been raped and sodomized since 1950 by clergy.

I cried as I digested these statistics. Finally, I reflected, however, that each person who is abused is just another person like me—a person whose body might store the trauma of certain memories in their tissues. A person whose brain might be easily triggered to interpret each new stimulus coming their way as danger, causing them to remain hyper-vigilant, hyper-aroused, on the verge of panic. I reflected that each person suffering from such trauma could benefit and heal, just as I did, from somatic therapy such as Margot's pelvic healing techniques that release energy stuck in the sexual tissues. Almost every relationship can benefit from tools like those we learned during Margot's training, tools that increase communication and intimacy, that encourage vulnerability and engender trust in one another.

I've learned, too, that just about every person has dark thoughts that could lead them astray—thoughts of self-hate, worthlessness—thoughts of shame and of being unlovable— thoughts that could keep them bound in victimhood. As such a person, I also know that anybody who commits to it can benefit from a practice of meditation, teaching them to direct attention and focus back to this precise moment, not leaning into the future, not falling into the past.

Whatever the circumstances, whatever has happened to them, anybody has the potential to heal from trauma and shame, anybody has the potential to experience more satisfying intimate relationships, *anybody*, whatever sacred or profane journey they have been on thus far, has the potential to experience mystical union.

To anyone out there searching for More, I recommend the resources listed in the "Further Reading" section.

Further Reading

Loving What Is, by Byron Katie
The Art of Sexual Ecstasy, by Margot Anand
The Four Agreements, by Don Miguel Ruiz
The Gift: Poems by Hafiz (tr. Daniel Ladinsky)
The Power of Now, by Eckhart Tolle
The Way of Selflessness, by Joel Morwood
There Is Nothing Wrong with You, by Cheri Huber
Zen Mind, Beginner's Mind, by Shunryu Suzuki

About the Author

Mariah lives in Alpine, California. She and her husband, Jake, frequently travel up and down the west coast from San Diego to Seattle for business and to visit family.

Mariah has raised two children, operated a freelance paralegal business, is a certified mediator, and has acted as Vice President of Corporate Communications for a high-technology business. She is also an awareness practitioner who has dedicated a significant portion of her life to exploring consciousness and ecstatic living. Mariah leads writing and meditation groups, classes and workshops in the greater San Diego area.

Visit www.sacredjourneytomore.com for periodic musings on life and the spiritual journey.

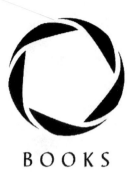

BOOKS

O is a symbol of the world, of oneness and unity; this eye represents knowledge and insight. We publish titles on general spirituality and living a spiritual life. We aim to inform and help you on your own journey in this life.

Visit our website: http://www.o-books.com

Find us on Facebook:
https://www.facebook.com/OBooks

Follow us on Twitter: @obooks